Containing Contagion

Containing Contagion

The Politics of Disease Outbreaks in Southeast Asia

SARA E. DAVIES

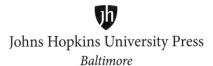

Johns Hopkins University Press

Baltimore

© 2019 Johns Hopkins University Press
All rights reserved. Published 2019
Printed in the United States of America on acid-free paper
9 8 7 6 5 4 3 2 1

Johns Hopkins University Press
2715 North Charles Street
Baltimore, Maryland 21218-4363
www.press.jhu.edu

Library of Congress Cataloging-in-Publication Data

Names: Davies, Sara Ellen, author.
Title: Containing contagion : the politics of disease outbreaks in Southeast Asia /
    Sara E. Davies.
Description: Baltimore : Johns Hopkins University Press, 2019. |
    Includes bibliographical references and index.
Identifiers: LCCN 2018027547 | ISBN 9781421427393 (pbk. : alk. paper) |
    ISBN 1421427397 (pbk. : alk. paper) | ISBN 9781421427409 (electronic) |
    ISBN 1421427400 (electronic)
Subjects: | MESH: ASEAN. | World Health Organization. | Communicable Disease
    Control—legislation & jurisprudence | Disease Outbreaks—prevention & control |
    Global Health | Health Policy | Health Services Administration | International
    Cooperation | International Agencies | Asia, Southeastern—epidemiology
Classification: LCC RA441 | NLM WA 33 JA25 | DDC 362.10959—dc23
LC record available at https://lccn.loc.gov/2018027547

A catalog record for this book is available from the British Library.

*Special discounts are available for bulk purchases of this book. For more information,
please contact Special Sales at 410-516-6936 or specialsales@press.jhu.edu.*

Johns Hopkins University Press uses environmentally friendly book materials,
including recycled text paper that is composed of at least 30 percent post-consumer
waste, whenever possible.

For Isaac
All my love always

CONTENTS

I am deeply grateful to Robin Coleman at Johns Hopkins University Press for his trust and faith in this book from the outset. Thank you, Juliana McCarthy and Hilary Jacqmin, for taking care of the manuscript to completion. Thanks to Carrie Watterson for her prodigious copyediting skill and Becky Hornyak for the index. I sincerely thank the reviewers who reviewed the proposal and the manuscript. I am grateful for their enthusiasm, their constructive criticism, and their attention to detail. Thank you, Adam Kamradt-Scott and Simon Rushton, for being so supportive when I suggested this book as a follow-up to our book.

Words cannot begin to convey my appreciation to the individuals who assisted me with their time, advice, and contacts to make this research project possible. The generosity I encountered in the region and beyond still takes my breath away. In my work, transcripts, documents, archives—but especially interviews—are my lifeline to understanding the world of international relations in action. First and foremost, a massive thank-you to individuals within the Association of Southeast Asian Nations (ASEAN) secretariat, and within the World Health Organization's regional offices and country offices for South-East Asia and the Western Pacific. The Communicable Disease Section/Unit in both regional offices were tremendously supportive. A big thank-you to the administrative teams in both offices who made sure my questions and requests for a meeting were always answered. I am sorry I cannot name everyone: some individuals wanted anonymity, and so I decided in fairness to make everyone anonymous. When you hold the copy I send to you, please know how grateful I am to you for making this project possible. I hope I have produced a volume of work that you will find honest and instructive.

Second, to individuals within the ministries of health from the ASEAN member states: I was greeted in every country with such warmth and hospitality. I am grateful to every person who treated my questions with such seriousness. Thank you to WHO headquarters for patiently providing me with a list of people to talk to as I began and, then again, as I closed this project. Thank you to individual members of the Asia Pacific Strategy for Emerging Diseases (APSED) Technical Advisory Group who generously talked to me at length about their work. Finally, thank you to the other international organizations and national governments for their assistance when I visited in-country and at events: the United Nations Development Programme, the World Bank, and federal-level public health and foreign affairs representatives from Australia, Papua New Guinea, Canada, China, Japan, New Zealand, South Korea, the United Kingdom, and the United States.

I am grateful to the Australian Research Council for generously supporting my work. I am especially grateful to Professor Hilary Charlesworth, who kindly read multiple versions of my first Australian Research Council grant. I received an Australian Postdoctoral Fellowship Award (DP0878792) and a Future Fellowship (FT1301040), both of which supported my research for this project. I am humbled by such generosity. I have also explored themes in this book in articles that may interest readers: "Mind the Human Rights Gap in Outbreak Response," *Medical Law Review* 25 (2) 2017; "Healthy Populations, Political Stability and Regime Type: Southeast Asia as a Case Study," *Review of International Studies* 40 (5) 2014; "The International Politics of Disease Reporting: Towards Post-Westphalianism?," *International Politics* 49 (5) 2012.

I thank my institution, Griffith University, especially the School of Government and International Relations, the Centre for Governance and Public Policy, and the Griffith Asia Institute. Thank you to my colleagues who patiently heard many versions presented of this book. Thank you to my research assistants who helped me with this project with such skill and dedication: Elliot Dolan-Evans, Naila Maier-Knapp, Troy O'Neill, Stephanie Pearson, and Dyonne Pennings.

Thank you, Belinda Bennett, Mely Caballero-Anthony, Stefan Elbe, Juanita Elias, Sophie Harman, Fiona McDonald, Anne Roemer-Mahler, Jacqui True, Clare Wenham, Wesley Widmaier, and Jeremy Youde.

Finally, all my love and appreciation to my family (Mum, Dad, Jane, Tony, Clair, and James). Alex, my best friend and husband, always constant and supportive. Thank you for making me laugh and keep things in perspective and for your endless faith in my abilities. I dedicate this book to my son, Isaac. Thank you for your patience when I was distracted, your kindness, your love, your strength, and your intelligence. You keep me centered. I dedicate this book to you with my deepest and eternal love.

Any errors in the book are mine alone.

AFRO	Regional Office for Africa
AHMM	ASEAN Health Ministers Meeting
AI	avian influenza
APSED	Asia Pacific Strategy for Emerging Infectious Diseases
APT	ASEAN Plus Three
ASEAN	Association of Southeast Asian Nations
CSR	Communicable Disease Surveillance and Response
DALY	Disability-Adjusted Life Year
DHF	dengue hemorrhagic fever
DON	*Disease Outbreak News*
EID	emerging infectious disease
EMRO	Regional Office for the Eastern Mediterranean
EURO	European Regional Office
FAO	Food and Agriculture Organization
GHO	Global Health Observatory
GHSA	Global Health Security Agenda
GISN	Global Influenza Surveillance Network
GISRS	Global Influenza Surveillance and Response System
GOARN	Global Outbreak Alert Response Network
GPHIN	Global Public Health Information Network
HALE	Health-Adjusted Life Expectancy
HPAI	highly pathogenic avian influenza
IHME	Institute for Health Metrics Evaluation
IHR	International Health Regulations
IR	international relations
ISR	International Sanitary Regulations
JE	Japanese encephalitis
JEE	Joint External Evaluation
MBDS	Mekong Basin Disease Surveillance
MERS	Middle East Respiratory Syndrome

NFP	National Focal Point
OIHP	Office International d'Hygiene Publique
PAHO	Pan American Health Organization
PASB	Pan American Sanitary Bureau
PHEIC	Public Health Emergency of International Concern
PMM	ProMED-mail / Program for Monitoring Emerging Diseases
SARS	severe acute respiratory syndrome
SEARO	South-East Asia Regional Office
TAC	Treaty of Amity and Cooperation
TAG EID	Technical Advisory Group for Emerging Infectious Diseases
TB	tuberculosis
UCDP	Uppsala Conflict Data Program
UPR	Universal Periodic Review
WER	*Weekly Epidemiological Report*
WHA	World Health Assembly
WHO	World Health Organization
WHO-SEAJPH	*WHO South East Asia Journal of Public Health*
WPRO	Western Pacific Regional Office
WPSAR	*Western Pacific Surveillance and Response Journal*

A Study of Southeast Asia's Response to Infectious Disease Outbreaks

Do states have a duty to prevent infectious disease outbreaks from spreading beyond their borders? Focusing on one of the world's most pivotal regions in the field of global health—Southeast Asia—in this book I examine the extent to which states have begun to recognize a duty to prevent the spread of diseases, how recognition of this duty has shaped practice, and the many challenges that still lie ahead.

The idea that states have a duty to prevent the spread of diseases by reporting outbreak events that may pose a Public Health Emergency of International Concern (PHEIC)[1] was included in the revised International Health Regulations (IHR) agreed to by states on 23 May 2005 (WHA 2005). The World Health Organization's (WHO) principal decision-making body, the World Health Assembly (WHA), which comprises all UN member states, agreed that all states should take action "to prevent, protect against, control and provide a public health response to the international spread of disease in ways that are commensurate with and restricted to public health risks." Since the revised IHR came into force in 2007, states have worked individually and collectively to meet the IHR's core capacity requirements to contain public health threats as defined under the new framework (Fischer and Katz 2013 153–156).

The revised IHR offered a "legal instrument [that seeks] to ensure global health security through a *collective approach*" (Li and Kasai 2011: 7; emphasis added). States agreed to share the duty to prevent, detect, and respond to major disease outbreaks by measuring their own performance against eight core capacities, by permitting non-state actors to inform the WHO of outbreaks, and by cooperating on the necessary responses, which may range from surveillance and response standards to laboratory processes, treatment, legislation, and risk communication (Plotkin and Hardiman 2013).

However, the path toward implementation of the IHR has not been smooth. Systemic weaknesses were most obviously exposed by the world's inadequate initial response to the 2014 Ebola outbreak in West Africa. Before that, however, outbreaks of various types of influenza in East Asia had tested the new norms to the limit (Stevenson and Cooper 2009; Elbe 2010). In 2009, the H1N1 influenza outbreak highlighted three critical tensions with its implementation.

First, there were unresolved questions about who, precisely, should guide states during an outbreak and through the process of following reporting procedure.

Second, questions arose about the coordination of communication flows (particularly when non-state actors report an outbreak to the WHO regional office or headquarters that the state itself denies). There were also questions posed about where responsibility begins and ends in situations where the affected state refuses to confirm an outbreak or confirm the extent of the outbreak. Resting on the assumption that transparency would satisfy the enlightened self-interest of states more than secrecy would, the revised IHR were meant to resolve this conundrum by encouraging states to report as responsible actors. In practice, however, the balance of interests between reporting and not reporting was not so clear. Despite recurrent claims that states would benefit directly by reporting early and often, practical experience suggests that early reporting could incur significant political and financial penalties (Kamradt-Scott 2016: 411). During the H1N1 and Ebola outbreaks, several countries imposed travel and trade sanctions against countries that reported infections, despite being urged not to (Davies, Kamradt-Scott, and Rushton 2015: chap. 5). Unsurprisingly, as a result, the fear remains that economic costs might encourage states to attempt to conceal an outbreak rather than openly report (Calain and Abu Sa'Da 2015).

Third, these experiences exposed questions about the normative capacity of the IHR to secure state compliance during outbreak emergencies. The IHR are a regulatory framework, not a convention. A convention must be formally signed and ratified by states, whereas the regulations impose no such legal obligation (Plotkin 2007: 840–845).

In an earlier book with Adam Kamradt-Scott and Simon Rushton, I explored the background, drafting, adoption, and implementation of the revised IHR as an example of international "disease diplomacy" (Davies, Kamradt-Scott, and Rushton 2015). In that volume, we focused on the international political processes that characterized the remaking of the global health security regime: the securitization of disease, in particular, the rise of the concept "global health security" that enabled (and in some ways constrained) political support for the IHR revision process. We identified and tracked the promotion of new behavioral expectations (norms) on states concerning their "obligation" to report outbreaks and the politics around the practical impediments to states fulfilling their IHR (2005) duties. Influenced by the "norm life cycle" model, we followed the passage of the revised IHR (and the new norms embodied therein) to see how it configured with the three stages of norm emergence (introduction of the norm), norm socialization (acceptance of the norm), and norm internalization (diffusion of the norm) (Finnemore and Sikkink 1998).

In this book, I turn to the question of internalization in one of the most significant and riskiest regions: Southeast Asia. I examine the extent to which states in the region have complied with the new regulations and the challenges that have arisen. In 2005, the same year the revised IHR were adopted, the Asia Pacific Strategy for Emerging Infectious Diseases (APSED) framework was created to run from 2005 to 2010; its objective was to assist states in the Asia and Pacific region to implement the revised regulations. A combination of regional political institutions (Association of Southeast Asian Nations [ASEAN] and ASEAN Plus Three [APT; Japan, China, and South Korea]), with technical international institutions (WHO South-East Asia Regional Office [SEARO], WHO Western Pacific Regional Office [WPRO], and WHO headquarters) facilitated regional cooperation that pushed Southeast Asian states closer to IHR compliance. By the end of APSED's first phase, many if not most Southeast Asian governments had come to recognize a duty to prevent the spread of infectious diseases across national borders. Through the deliberate alignment of political interest and regional cooperation with the achievement of the technical capacity to detect and report, the Southeast Asian experience provides important insight on how to begin collective realization of a duty to report outbreak events.

The Regional Case for the IHR

Immediately after the adoption of the IHR by the WHA in 2005, member states in the WHO's regional groupings for Southeast Asia[2] and the Western Pacific[3] began meeting to develop a collective strategy for addressing emerging infectious disease outbreaks. The result was the APSED framework, which was adopted in September 2005 by member states of both SEARO and the WPRO at their respective regional assemblies (WPRO 2005). APSED was meant to provide a "common strategic framework for the countries and areas of the region to build sustainable national and regional capacities and partnerships in the Asia Pacific region" (Kumaresan and Huikuri 2015: 60). What is more, in the years that followed, ASEAN member states and the APT grouping contributed their own collaborative processes focused on strengthening emerging infectious disease preparedness in line with the IHR and APSED (Caballero-Anthony 2008).

Southeast Asian states, aligned through their ASEAN membership, are especially committed to the principle of noninterference concerning the domestic affairs of sovereigns (Gerard 2013). Given the region's long-standing commitment to noninterference, the member states' decision to acquiesce to an international regulation coupled with a framework that permitted evaluations, even interference and judgment, from an international organization, the WHO, is curious. Moreover, regional acceptance of the IHR contradicted behavior from the same member states that had opposed similar demands for acceptance of international norms in other areas (i.e., civil and political human rights, refugee status recognition) (Acharya 2007; Collins 2013; M. Davies 2013; Gerard 2013). As I explore in the book, the pursuit of capacity-building goals as a *cooperative* endeavor—despite the different political, social, and technical challenges they face—was a unique response from the region.

ASEAN member states, despite vastly different health system capacities and political systems, agreed to pursue a collective approach for the communication of outbreak events. As this book reveals through data and interview analysis, ASEAN member states consistently pursued and acted upon cooperative arrangements after the adoption of the IHR in 2005. These arrangements were largely associated with and supported by the aforementioned APSED, which prioritized particular core capacities for phased implementation in the region. The focus in this book is on the political cooperation forged during APSED's first phase, 2005–2010, and its particular emphasis on surveillance as an achievable and desirable goal for beginning the process of meeting IHR core capacities (Ijaz et al. 2012: 1054–1057).[4] Explaining why ASEAN states adopted a collective approach, the complications of this collective approach, and the consequences of this approach for IHR implementation, is the key aim of this book.

The Curious Case of ASEAN

This book examines how one region—10 Southeast Asian states that are members of ASEAN—engaged with the revised IHR while responding to a wave of emerging and endemic infectious disease outbreaks in the first decade of the twenty-first century. Those outbreaks range from Nipah to severe acute respiratory syndrome (SARS) and H5N1, to dengue and Japanese encephalitis (JE). I examine how a region of states with very different domestic institutional capacities and political environments has responded to the tensions between the demands of IHR implementation and its cherished principle of noninterference. I look at how and why this regional organization worked in cooperation with the WHO WPRO and the WHO SEARO, through APSED, to create deep patterns of informal regional cooperation to meet the IHR core capacity requirements. I explore a decade of disease outbreak reporting between the WHO organization and ASEAN member states to reveal significant behavior change in outbreak notification of disease events—both within and among these states, as well as in their reporting behavior to WHO. I argue that this was a decade of deliberate epistemic (technical knowledge-focused) community building involving technical (health) experts, political actors (ASEAN representatives from member states), and WHO staff (from headquarters and regional offices) (Haas 1992). Regular face-to-face meetings on matters concerning each of the eight core capacities progressed local adaption of the IHR and created opportunities to meaningfully adapt the IHR to local circumstances (Acharya 2004; Sandholtz 2008).

Some actors played especially important roles in this process. I show how the ASEAN secretariat's Health Division and individuals within the WHO WPRO and SEARO acted as normative champions and devoted considerable effort to raising awareness of the IHR and its core capacity requirements among states through these epistemic communities. ASEAN itself played an important and, as yet, underexamined role. Its role underscores the need to include actors beyond WHO headquarters, to give WHO regional offices tangible responsibility for programs devoted to IHR compliance, and to confront the political environment in which individual states must practice IHR implementation. In the case of Southeast Asia, its primary regional organization and networks outside the WHO played a politically important role in facilitating normative and technical knowledge transfer between states and the WHO to implement the IHR.[5]

This book's argument is a controversial one. I present ASEAN as a community of states that can promote compliance and conformity to international rules in spite of its diverse membership. This view runs counter to some international relations (IR) scholarship on ASEAN regionalism (Narine 2002; Jones 2012) and recent discussion on ASEAN normative evolution concerning matters such as human rights and socioeconomic commitments (Haacke and Williams 2008; Collins 2013; Gerard 2013; M. Davies 2013). It is a view that may be challenged by some analysts of health governance in the region (Lee and Fidler 2007; Yoon 2010; Coker et al. 2011; Lamy and Phua 2012; Kamradt-Scott, Lee, and Xu 2013; Hameiri 2014). Most accounts of ASEAN and its role in promoting health cooperation in Southeast Asia, particularly around disease outbreak response, hold that the grouping inspires only thin, mainly instrumental and rhetorical, cooperation that drives only minimal institutional and behavioral change at the regional or domestic level.

These views contend that the lack of formal legislative and funding mechanisms, along with dependence on elite political relationships to progress reform, make ASEAN a weak institutional body for promoting change. In looking at health cooperation practices in ASEAN, much of the analysis is informed by a "benchmark" of formal institutionalism where ASEAN, as a regional institution, is compared to other regional organizations (Maier-Knapp 2011; Amaya, Rollet, and Kingah 2015). However, ASEAN's formal institutions are only one dimension of how the regional organization achieves cooperation and compliance from member states (Acharya 2009; Murray 2014). It has been argued that Southeast Asia's form of association must be judged on its own terms (Leifer 1989: 119; Tarling 2006: 4). Here is a group of states whose association is characterized by informal, dense networks that are as important as the formal institutions when it comes to influencing the behavior of members states (Arase 2010; Johnston 2012; Goh 2014).

This scholarship argues for attention to be paid to how ASEAN confronts threats and responds at the institutional *and* normative level (Acharya 2009). Cooperation in ASEAN is at its strongest when leadership agrees to unite on a particular (security-centered) issue (Ba 2010; Stubbs 2014). This contemporary analysis has observed that ASEAN can and has achieved compliance, coherence, and strength from informal interactions (Caballero-Anthony and Emmers 2006; Ba 2010). Furthermore, it would be wrong to presume that the evolution of ASEAN's formal institutions is not taking place and not having a serious influence on the interaction of its member states (Haacke and Morada 2010).

In 2009, ASEAN member states agreed to a formal legal institutional arrangement to pursue greater regional cooperation in economic and security matters—the ASEAN Charter (ASEAN 2008). The same charter also agreed to the "seminal" inclusion of a human rights mechanism (the ASEAN Intergovernmental Commission on Human Rights) (Tan 2011: 4). The growth of mechanisms such as the ASEAN Intergovernmental Commission on Human Rights and the ASEAN Committee on Women and Children, and the interconnectedness of these bodies with ASEAN's "traditional" focus—political and security, economic and sociocultural pillars—has created the opportunity for normative and domestic institutional change through expanded networks that identify new security threats that require new forms of cooperation and collective action (Caballero-Anthony 2014).

In this book I am guided by this contemporary scholarship on ASEAN, which has highlighted the normative role played by the regional body as a "discursive vehicle for the collective articulation of space, engendered by shared norms and identify, and cooperative action" devised to manage cooperation within an order whose rules are established by others (Goh 2013: 120). ASEAN's contribution, as a regional institution, comes from the adoption and adaption of international norms to local contexts and realities (Acharya 2009: 144). As such, the theoretical framework that underpins this book is attention to normative engagements as a tool to promote diplomatic collaboration and transparency. Specifically, under what conditions does shared identity give rise to create functional cooperation between governments and, through this, create networks of epistemic communities that influence one another (Ba 2009: 4)? Informed by prior normative studies of ASEAN (Acharya 2009; Tan 2011; Caballero-Anthony 2014), I find that the more ASEAN states commit to (informal) consensus statements on core capacities around the IHR—in particular, surveillance and reporting disease outbreaks—the more they appeared to drive important behavioral changes at the national level where executive function, budget, and legislation must adapt to keep up with the regional pace. While ASEAN's formal institutions may be underdeveloped, the informal networks that underlie them are robust.

This study does not argue that every Southeast Asian state has achieved perfect compliance. The internalization of necessary political reform to meet the IHR revisions will continue to be challenging in some domestic environments. I identify significant and ongoing state-level political barriers to IHR implementation that exist in addition to technical and health system capacity shortfalls. In light of these obstacles, what contribution does regional cooperation facilitate? The APSED framework gave permission to those working within the parameters of the noninterference principle to step outside it to strengthen the sovereign in addressing health security: health ministries and the officials within them working on infectious disease response collaborate, share, and debate—sometimes weekly—with their counterparts in other member states. In the presence of centralized, sometimes authoritarian, political structures, these dense networks offer opportunities to instantiate shared expectations and encourage behavioral change.

I present a story of a revised IHR that is being locally adapted in Southeast Asia to meet the political, social, and technical needs of states as they modify their behavior to carry out the reporting and response duties specified by the instrument. As this book will detail, these adaptions are not perfect, but their promise comes from the attention paid to relationships among health officials within the ASEAN collective and personal relationships between the ASEAN secretariat and the SEARO and WPRO regional offices. From the exchange of staff to the regular program of workshops and conferences, compliance pull is achieved through informal processes, where pilot study results, budgetary obstacles, and ministerial dilemmas are shared over lunches, dinners, and small breakout sessions. Information about expectations, progress, and challenges is shared through frequent face-to-face dialogue and direct interaction between officials.

This is a story focused primarily on the formal and informal exchanges over IHR compliance between 2005 and 2010. At this time the Southeast Asian region was under tremendous pressure from and observation by the international community. The region had been the center of the SARS outbreak in 2003, swiftly followed by an avian influenza (AI) outbreak that was creating public panic and wreaking havoc on farmers and the poultry industry across the region, when the revised IHR were adopted in 2005. This book charts why emphasis at this fragile time was to join the regional and the local: to create personal networks.

The normative approach and practice adopted in Asia speaks to the approach being adopted by WHO headquarters in the wake of the catastrophic Ebola outbreak. The WHO's 2016 Health Emergencies Programme appears to have learned the lessons of Ebola by streamlining reporting and accountability lines. Under the new guidance, country offices are to report directly to WHO headquarters (WHO 2016a). Coupled with this effort to centralize IHR reporting is renewed emphasis on joint evaluations of states' IHR core capacities by external actors. Donor funding and evaluations focus on country performance. These reforms are a deliberate step away from the regionalized and self-reporting approach adopted initially after 2005, which countries had been permitted up until the Ebola outbreak crisis. This book serves as a cautionary tale in response to these trends and makes an argument for identifying regionalism as one of multiple pathways to implement the IHR. Regional engagement in outbreak response, as well as self-reporting functions, is an important tool for localizing and adapting the IHR to regional concerns and for changing actual behavior. IHR implementation is first and foremost not a technical exercise but a political one that requires political ownership and commitment to make it work. This ownership is sustained, in large part, by the dense regional networks facilitated by ASEAN and APSED. Moves toward centralization and bilateral performance measures could, in some politically fragile environments wary of imposed benchmarks, make implementation of the IHR more, not less, difficult.

Book Outline

The book unfolds in six chapters. In chapter 1, I present a brief history of the adoption of the revised IHR in 2005 and the effort to implement the IHR core capacities among the 190-odd member states of the World Health Assembly since the instrument came into force in 2007. The chapter explores three dominant narratives that have emerged since then about the IHR and their implementation.[6] These narratives began to emerge after WHO director-general Margaret Chan's first declaration of a PHEIC in response to the H1N1 "swine flu" outbreak in 2009, and they have grown in prominence after the belated PHEIC declaration by WHO in response to the Ebola outbreak in West Africa in 2014 (Gostin and Katz 2016).

The first is that the WHO's decentralized structure inhibits accountability for the implementation of the IHR core capacities. The second is that, because of these structural tensions and the designation of the instrument as a regulation rather than treaty, states do not take the IHR instrument as seriously in the areas that required enhanced compliance, such as following WHO-recommended trade and travel measures, as well as consistent monitoring and evaluation of IHR core capacities, followed up with annual reports to the WHO (these are the common noncompliance areas raised). The third, related to the second, is that the absence of a funding mechanism to support the investments needed to build IHR core capacities inhibits low- and middle-income states from taking the steps necessary to comply with their duties in the context of their already financially and administratively pressurized health system environment. I consider how these arguments have shaped contemporary engagement with the progress of the revised IHR and how the post-Ebola reviews of the IHR have, overall, presented a largely negative picture of member states' progress in implementing the IHR. I argue that most studies on the IHR tend to focus on the failings of the instrument (e.g., the often quoted "two-thirds of states have failed to meet the IHR core capacities"; Moon et al. 2015: 2209). Curiously, however, little attention has been devoted to the areas and locations of progress since 2005, despite what I argue are clear signs of progress. Two regions in particular where consistent gains were made upon the adoption of the IHR revisions were the states that sit in WHO regional offices of the Western Pacific and Southeast Asia.

In the second chapter I examine the context of Southeast Asia more closely. Southeast Asian states shared affinity in being primarily affected by the SARS and H5N1 avian influenza outbreak at the time of the IHR revision and adoption. Yet, in their individual capability to adopt the revised IHR core capacity requirements, they were vastly different. In this chapter, I argue that, to understand the conditions necessary for IHR compliance, we need to tell not just a technical story but a political one as well. It is vital to attend to the political context in which IHR implementation must occur in order to understand how behaviors change and how actors balance competing priorities and concerns. Here I examine the ASEAN region's underlying political difficulties and conditions that make IHR compliance difficult to achieve. A region with a tradition of resistance to international standards coupled with a normative commitment to noninterference are not the best conditions for encouraging a shared duty to report disease outbreak events. This is what makes Southeast Asia such an important case.

In the third chapter, I provide a more detailed account of the pressure that the Southeast Asian region was under at the time of the revised IHR. Here, I focus in particular on SARS in Singapore and Viet Nam in 2003 and the outbreak of H5N1 in late 2004 and early 2005 with human infections in Cambodia, Indonesia, Laos, Thailand, and Viet Nam. I argue that the region's experience as a disease "hot zone" (Jones et al. 2008) coupled with the immense political reforms taking place in ASEAN at the time of these disease outbreaks, saw rather dramatic health governance reforms in-country, which meant that the region was actually positively disposed toward a regional framework for implementing the revised IHR to improve both state and regional resilience to disease outbreak events. The timing was immensely important: the ASEAN secretariat and WHO seized upon it. In this chapter I argue that a normative change was taking place among ASEAN's membership. Security threats were being appreciated as *collective* threats to regional security, as opposed to the earlier lens of viewing traditional security threats solely as threats to the sovereign. "Nontraditional" security threats in particular were taking hold in the region and shaping practices (Caballero-Anthony 2014). The introduction of the term "health security" into the regional lexicon created a political environment of readiness to introduce reforms necessary to inhibit the spread of disease. It also helped overcome the potential for individual affected states to be stigmatized. This collective approach to health security—a view that held that individual states were only strong if they acted through collective approaches to health governance reform—was vital and timely in creating a positive regional response to the revised IHR.

In the fourth chapter, I detail the creation of APSED, a regional engagement mechanism to promote the revised IHR in Southeast Asia and beyond. APSED was a framework developed in specific recognition that the Asia Pacific region has a diverse range of low-, middle-, and high-income countries with different public health system capacities that would need to adapt to the IHR core capacities in ways that accommodated their different levels of competence and existing capacity. One of the areas emphasized in APSED was the need to implement the IHR not only nationally but regionally. This focus on the regional dimension stood at odds with the approach taken by WHO headquarters. There, the emphasis was placed firmly on national-level and international-level responsibility. The APSED framework was presented as a "middle path" that articulated a regional risk of disease outbreaks that required regional cooperation. This regional framing of global health security was, I argue, unique to the region and an essential part of diffusing the revised IHR. This tripartite relationship among the member state, the ASEAN secretariat, and the WHO regional office(s) was different from other arrangements in place for IHR implementation at the time. It helped localize the IHR and mitigate the potential normative clash between these regulations and the region's principle of noninterference.

To appreciate how APSED affected ASEAN, we need to have baseline knowledge of ASEAN member states' behavior in the area of public notification of disease outbreaks—a clearest indication of capacity is in the area of outbreak detection and reporting. In chapter 5 I chart the disease outbreak reporting behavior of ASEAN member states from 1996 to 2010. The year 1996 was just prior to the outbreak of Nipah virus in Malaysia in 1998 and a large outbreak of dengue fever in the same year. I follow outbreak-reporting trends up to 2010, the first year that states were formally invited to report to the WHO director-general their progress in meeting the IHR core capacities and the end of APSED's first phase. I trace each state's reports to the WHO, which were documented in the weekly, then daily outbreak news service, and I trace media reports (which include government notices) of outbreak events to compare individual countries' reporting performance to the WHO with the volume of disease outbreak events in each country. I compare reporting behavior for novel disease outbreak outbreaks with endemic disease outbreaks like encephalitis and dengue fever. This chapter reveals that ASEAN states' reporting practice of disease outbreak events—even the most recalcitrant—changed under the normative influence of the APSED framework. The analysis also reveals the importance of understanding why there is differentiation in states' reporting practices.

In chapter 6, I consider what explanations may account for the different ways in which ASEAN states individually manage their disease outbreak alerts. Informed by the dataset presented in chapter 5, it is true that all states experienced an upward trend in reporting practices, but reporting "black holes," those situations where disease outbreaks were occurring but the affected state was not reporting, remain. In this chapter I consider how we interpret reporting black holes. How significant is it for states to report suspected disease outbreaks rather than laboratory confirmed disease outbreaks? How do we judge a country's poor reporting performance: does this suggest a resourcing and capacity shortfall or deliberate political interference in the reporting process? Supported by qualitative interviews and access to internal documentation in the region, I attempt to understand the reporting behaviors that evolved during APSED's first phase and what response has evolved after the first phase to address different reporting patterns.

In the conclusion I detail the significant obstacles to IHR implementation that remain. I contend that these obstacles are political as much as they are technical. As such, the importance of regional forums is that they provide a shared venue to express concerns among like-minded states and, at the same time, encourage solutions to address these concerns. Bilateral donor programs and assessment exercises serve in providing specific, technical advice, but they rarely provide the "cover" needed for a frank exchange. APSED achieved consensus among all states, even the most recalcitrant, that meeting the IHR revisions is important for individual and collective health security. Within this region no state has (yet) argued that it has no responsibility to promptly and transparently report disease outbreak events to its neighboring states. This is a significant shift in how ASEAN states view the applicability of the noninterference norm when it comes to disease outbreak events and their collective responsibility to disease outbreak reporting. APSED provided a framework to translate the ambitions of WHO headquarters, and ASEAN provided the normative language to translate those ambitions on the ground in Southeast Asia. Relationships within programs like APSED and APT Emerging Infectious Diseases (EID) Programme provided safe venues to hear and voice obstacles under a veil of relative confidentiality in a forum where states understood the political as well as the technical capacity hurdles.

My inquiry points to the importance of regionally tailored IHR implementation programs like APSED. Such frameworks provide a narrative that is tailored to regional politics and experiences to come to grips with the capacities required under the revised IHR. The regional model assisted in the three specific ways: first, by establishing a mutually supportive regional context based on cherished regional principles (noninterference, avoidance of public criticism, etc.); second, by facilitating the emergence of dense networks of epistemic communities; and, third, by establishing a sense that the region confronted a common threat and had a shared regional responsibility to contain it.

Of course, capacity shortfalls and disagreements abounded. These shortfalls remain a concern and should be considered in any broader discussion of lessons learned from APSED. Identification of a shared threat and a shared responsibility does not mean there is a shared capacity. However, the Southeast Asian experience provides important lessons about the broader processes of securing IHR compliance from different countries, in different regions, with different capacities. In particular, it points to the need to look beyond the promotion of technical capacity-building measures and to also invest in regional organizations that encourage the creation of shared norms and informal networks.

CHAPTER ONE

The Revised International
Health Regulations in Practice

The revised International Health Regulations were adopted at the Fifty-Eighth World Health Assembly on 23 May 2005. The original IHR (formerly called the International Sanitary Regulations) had been adopted by the WHA in 1951. The IHR, from their inception, have been concerned with the control of infectious disease outbreaks by states adopting procedures at ports of entry (air, land, and sea). In 1969, the instrument was renamed the IHR and its alert function for six diseases was reduced to four diseases (cholera, plague, smallpox, or yellow fever; typhus and relapsing fever were removed).

The purpose of the IHR is twofold: to establish a framework through which states can notify the international community of disease outbreak events and to provide advice and technical assistance to states on public health safety measures at land, sea, and airports (check passports to confirm yellow fever vaccinations, permission to de-rat ships, etc.). Amendments to the 1969 IHR at the 1973 WHA and 1983 WHA, coupled with the successful eradication of the smallpox, reduced the IHR coverage to three diseases: cholera, plague, and yellow fever. States were always expected to report confirmed outbreak events of these three diseases and comply with the WHO's recommendations on the trade, travel, and vaccination (for yellow fever). The WHO would provide a public record of outbreak notices in its weekly epidemiological report and confirm when the outbreak was over, if it was notified by the state.

By the mid-1990s this framework was becoming increasingly strained. States were not always reporting outbreaks of these three diseases, and when reports were made available the weekly updates were often too late to assist neighboring states with their response. The WHO provided no recommendations on the detection and reporting of new infectious diseases that could pose significant risk to populations (e.g., Ebola hemorrhagic fever), the WHO director-general had limited means by which to encourage states to improve their surveillance and detection procedures, and the WHO did not have authority to independently verify and report disease outbreaks without the affected state's permission. States that did not want it known, for example, that they regularly experienced cholera outbreaks chose not to report (Fidler 2004a: 34). Recognizing these flaws in the system, in 1995 the WHA adopted Resolution 48.7, calling for the WHO director-general to revise the IHR, specifically, to convene a committee to engage in regional consultations to develop a new reporting and detection model for the IHR. In addition to the revision discussion, the WHO was arguing for an improvement to the quality of surveillance information: "WHO's proposal to replace the IHR's limited disease coverage with duties to report the broader category of 'public health emergencies of international concern' would combine with a larger supply of information to improve global surveillance data as a public good . . . Furthermore, the proposal on use of non-governmental information proved the most compelling IHR revision idea. The potential of transforming international surveillance into global surveillance as envisioned in the IHR revision process was so substantial that WHO began to harvest it early in the process" (Fidler 2004a: 66).

Consultations and model testing followed for the next eight years. There was a glimmer of the potential revision that the WHO sought when its use of nongovernmental sources of surveillance information was approved in the 2001 WHA (Fidler 2004a: 67): the Canadian-based Global Public Health Intelligence Network (GPHIN) search engine had been in use by WHO headquarters in its search for rumors and reports of disease events from around the world since 1998 (Grein et al. 2000). However, it was not until 2003 when an outbreak took on rapid global spread, a new viral respiratory disease of zoonotic origin called severe acute respiratory syndrome (SARS), that the WHA proposed an expedited two-year time frame for the negotiation of a final IHR text for adoption by May 2005. In May 2005, the WHA member states unanimously approved WHA Resolution 58.3: Revision of the International Health Regulations (WHA 2005).

The adoption of the revised IHR in 2005 has been the subject of much discussion in public health, international law, and international relations scholarship (inter alia, Fidler 2005, Zacher and Keefe 2008; Giorgetti 2012; Kamradt-Scott 2015). The revised IHR is a substantially different technical and political instrument from its antecedents. This was repeatedly stressed by delegates to the WHA meeting who adopted it (Whelan 2008) and by scholars since (see Katz and Fischer 2010; Gostin and Katz 2016). The claim that the revised IHR is "substantively" different from its earlier versions is demonstrated by the new requirements they impose on states (Fidler 2005: 358) and the values the revised IHR promoted (Zacher and Keefe 2008: 67). The revised IHR applied across the board and not just to a circumscribed list of specific diseases, in extreme cases the WHO director-general had authority to report on disease events without the permission of the affected state, and states agreed to meet eight core capacity requirement standards designed to enable them to better detect and report the broad category of health hazards that now fell under the revised IHR (in Annex 2). Moreover, in the revised IHR "states are called upon to also promote human rights, environmental protection, and security as well as the original two goals"[1] (Zacher and Keefe 2008: 67).

It has been commonly argued that the successful negotiation of the revised IHR was a significant diplomatic coup for the WHO, yet the regulations are also perceived as having failed to live up to their promise (Moon et al. 2015; Gostin and Katz 2016). The perceived failure of the revised IHR to sufficiently alter state behavior on disease outbreak response and containment has been attributed to three limitations: (1) the WHO's decentralized structure, which has no central authority to steer IHR implementation at the state level; (2) the IHR's perceived status (by states) as voluntary regulations rather than international legal obligations; and, (3) the absence of a funding mechanism to support states in building the core capacities. This chapter offers a brief history of the revised IHR and then turns in more depth to the three common perceptions outlined above. These contemporary understandings of the revised IHR suggest that the regulations have struggled to influence state practice, but these perceptions are only part of the lived story of the IHR.

The Revised IHR: A Brief History

The origins of the IHR date back to the mid-nineteenth century, when a cholera epidemic was spreading across Europe, mirroring the trade routes from Asia and the Middle East. Waves of cholera epidemics (three between 1830 and 1851) coupled with a desire to continue unimpeded trade led to the first international sanitary conference, held in Paris in 1851 (Fidler 1999: 27). For six months, 12 delegations, with a doctor and a diplomat attached to each country, discussed what form the convention should take, without coming to an agreement (Kamradt-Scott 2014: 191). Disagreements persisted for decades until the 10th such meeting, held in 1892, produced the first International Sanitary Convention (Heymann and West 2014: 101). Between 1892 and 1946,[2] there were 14 international sanitary meetings and 12 further agreements (Fidler 2005: 332; Kamradt-Scott 2014). These meetings and conventions, argues Kelley Lee, produced a form of "international health cooperation [that] reflected the concerns of the major European powers, namely to prevent epidemic diseases from disrupting their political and economic interests at home and abroad" (2008: 6). The agreements largely focused on surveillance and reporting, rather than on disease prevention and control at the source. This was the purpose of international cooperation on disease outbreak response, and the International Sanitary Convention facilitated no more than an orderly process for reporting disease outbreaks and suggesting appropriate quarantine responses.

Yet, despite these limitations, the International Sanitary Convention bequeathed three crucial things to global health security (Fidler 2005). First, it posited the idea that states should communicate and report outbreaks to an international institution or bureaucracy. The Sanitary Convention gave rise to the creation of the Office International d'Hygiene Publique (OIHP; France) in 1907 and the creation of the Pan American Sanitary Bureau in 1902 (PASB; North America). Both sanitary bureaus coordinated cooperation between the Americas and Europe concerning disease outbreak reporting under the International Sanitary Convention. Second, it established the principle of cooperation on disease reporting and quarantine standards at borders and ports (of entry) for three diseases, cholera, plague, and yellow fever, with the expectation that all travelers would carry vaccination/notification certificates. Third, it gave rise to the idea of a global organization for health. The League of Nations Health Organization, created after World War I, was given responsibility to circulate "epidemiological intelligence" and to compile reports of disease outbreaks that would inform the OIHP and the PASB (Brown, Cueto, and Fee 2006). The League of Nations Health Organization enjoyed relatively unimpeded access to states and colonial territories to gather and report disease outbreaks (via the colonies), produce annual statistical health yearbooks, and take an active role in circulating epidemic intelligence (disease outbreaks) and biostatistical data (Borowy 2009: 37–40). There is no doubt that the League's Health Organization served as an early institutional example for the WHO.

The creation of the League of Nations Health Organization in 1920 expanded international engagement on infectious diseases beyond the original focus of containment at European and North American borders (Borowy 2009). However, this was primarily driven by self-interest: "[Colonial] states realized that to balance disease protection and economic interests would require international cooperation and rules to reduce the friction and imbalance these goals produced. Thus, the earliest strategy taken by States was harmonization of quarantine [through the International Sanitary Convention]" (Fidler 1999: 52). Harmonized quarantine and advances in national public health systems removed some of the urgency for international diplomacy, but assistance would need to be directed to less-developed countries and regions to help their governments improve public health capabilities (Fidler 1999: 53).

At the end of World War II, focus on infectious disease surveillance and international reporting was preserved under the rubric of the new World Health Organization. Locating the International Sanitary Conventions under the WHO would give it one home—rather than managing notifications across three organizations in the PASB, OIHP, and the (now-defunct) League of Nations. With the adoption of the WHO Constitution in 1948 and the creation of a headquarters in Geneva and six regional offices (Americas, Africa, Europe, Middle East and North America, South-East Asia, and Western Pacific), the International Sanitary Regulations (ISR) were the first legal instrument adopted by WHO's member states' governing body, the World Health Assembly, in 1951 (Hardiman 2012).

The choice by WHA member states of a regulation rather than treaty—something retained in 2005—points to the idiosyncrasy of how member states saw the political function of the WHO as less important than its technical scientific function. Under Article 21 of the WHO Constitution, the WHA may adopt regulations without the need for states to annually report to the WHO director-general on their implementation (or failure to be implemented). Combined with the powers in Article 22, a regulation was an instrument that all WHA member states were expected to automatically recognize and adopt as members of the WHA, yet they were not themselves considered binding international law capable of imposing legal obligations upon states.[3]

States are entitled to "opt out" of the duties set out in the regulations by offering a submission and explanation to the WHA (Fidler 1999: 59–60). Optimists argued that this would allow states to implement the regulations immediately rather than having to wait for a requisite number of states to ratify before coming into force. The politics was assumed to be null and void. International sanitary *regulations* were proposed not because proponents believed that they could not successfully negotiate a convention but because regulations could be more readily expedited, more extensive, and more adaptable. In fact, the expectation at the time was that a broad range of regulations concerning health cooperation and access among member states would be adopted by the WHA in the early years (Taylor 2002).[4] Given the importance of preventing infectious disease outbreaks, it was assumed that an administratively weaker but more rapid and universal instrument would serve the desired purpose: facilitate the detection and reporting of disease outbreaks listed under the ISR. The more flexible regulations permitted the WHO director-general to seek WHA permission to update the inclusion or exclusion of a new disease, rather than having to go through the laborious process of renegotiating a treaty every time adjustments had to be made. Thus, it was assumed public health systems would be better served by regulations that could keep up with medical science and with new disease outbreaks. The reality, as Fidler (1999) presents in his historical analysis of the progression of international law concerning infectious disease control, is that in practice WHO headquarters found it difficult to update the regulations as regularly as necessary to be an effective public health tool. The WHA was no less politically divided than the UN Security Council and the UN General Assembly during the 1960s through the end of the Cold War (Chorev 2012). Resolutions were not easily passed in the WHA, which affected the development and application of broader IHR.

Reporting disease outbreak events to WHO headquarters was sporadic and unpredictable; while for those states that suffered with regular cholera and yellow fever outbreaks (in particular), the cost and consequence of reporting was burdensome. States persistently treated the regulations as a nonbinding instrument they could ignore with little to no political repercussions (Fidler 1999: 60–61). The principle of the regulations providing maximum security with minimum interference on trade and travel was not realized. States could be punitive with trade (to gain advantage) when a neighboring state reported, for example, cholera outbreaks in seafood or a plague outbreak in a village near an air- or seaport (Cash and Narasimhan 2000).

Yet it would be incorrect to state that the instrument had no demonstrable impact on the behavior of states (Giorgetti 2010: 85–86). All countries recognized and adopted the WHO-issued regulations concerning certification for yellow fever vaccination. This remains in place today. Similar procedures were established for smallpox, prior to its eradication in 1980. In both instances, there is no record of states challenging or flouting vaccination entry requirements attached to the IHR (Fluss and Gutteridge 1990). In the early years, irrespective of health system capacity, state-level procedures on infectious disease notification, vaccination, and disease eradication were implemented as a universal "commonsense" expectation and often reflected the content of the WHO's regulations (Bashford 2006). However, the IHR's circumscribed list of diseases and the tools available to contain these diseases became irrelevant and outdated as they were overtaken by state practice, the improvement of technologies, and the emergence of new diseases. There was also the persistent difficulty that states that did report disease outbreaks were often subjected to punitive, and economically damaging, restrictions by their neighbors, creating powerful disincentives to report (Cash and Narasimhan 2000).

Over time, the WHO division responsible for communicable disease came to the view that disease outbreaks were not being reported to headquarters; compromising the accuracy of reports in the WHO *Weekly Epidemiological Record* and increasing the number of outbreaks left unaddressed and thus susceptible to being spread across borders. It came to be taken for granted that the caseload and outbreak events in the weekly report were not accurate representations of the extent of outbreaks (Briggs and Mantini-Briggs 2003). Responsibility for reporting on the outbreak of three diseases (yellow fever, plague, and cholera) had grown from 60 countries in the 1950s to 170-plus countries by the 1990s, coupled with a reporting process that remained a weekly communication by fax and publication in a hard-copy report, which made the process increasingly anachronistic. The IHR instrument was not progressing with health technologies, changes in disease epidemiology, or the political reality of a growing WHA membership. There had been a dramatic geographic shift in membership at the World Health Assembly from the 1950s to the 1990s. In the early years the institutes of "colonial" and "tropical" medicine still had multiple locations across former empires that supplied outbreak information and pathology back to their respective headquarters—the London School of Tropical Medicine, the Pasteur Institute, or the Johns Hopkins Medical School—which would in turn be delivered to the WHO (Bashford 2006: 4). As decolonization gathered pace in the 1960s and 1970s, new ministries of public health and national universities emerged that wanted to collect and control their own outbreak information. The WHO's sources during this time changed, and the calculated benefit of reporting changed.

Finally, in 1995, the World Health Assembly agreed to revise the IHR (WHA Resolution 48.7) on the grounds that revision was needed to take "effective account of the threat posed by the international spread of new and re-emerging diseases" (WHA 1995). The IHR had reached their breaking point. The combination of the end of the Cold War and outbreak events including an outbreak of bubonic plague in Gujarat, India, in 1994 and Ebola in Kikwit, Democratic Republic of Congo (then Zaire), in 1995, had finally delivered political momentum among member states to address these limits (Fidler 1999: 65). The IHR had remained limited to specific disease coverage (cholera, plague, and yellow fever); by the 1990s this narrow application made the regulations increasingly irrelevant in the face of a predicted rise of novel and reemerging novel infectious diseases. The detection of drug-resistant tuberculosis (TB) and new hemorrhagic fevers (including Ebola), coupled with the prediction of an "inevitable" pandemic influenza, were matched with equal concern that the fall of the Soviet Union would lead to the spread of laboratory-grown bio-weapons being sold on the black market (Enemark 2007; Koblentz 2012). For all these scenarios, the existing IHR had no mandate to report on or provide advice. The instrument was primarily an extension of the reporting practice established at the turn of the twentieth century (Fidler 1999: 64). Coupled with its lack of incentives to encourage compliance, the stated aim of the 1969 IHR—to routinize reporting to facilitate minimum interference with travel and trade— belied the fact that many states thought their national interest was best achieved by concealing an outbreak from the WHO (Cash and Narasimhan 2000).

What triggered greater political attention to the ineffectiveness of the IHR in the 1990s? The political climate within the WHA reflected the broader environment of diplomatic cooperation and negotiation across the UN at the end of the Cold War (Taylor 2002; Whelan 2008). Interest in reforming the regulations, and the possibility that consensus might be found, reflected broader developments across the UN system of giving greater attention to the human (in)security conditions that prolong economic and political fragility in states and regions (Thakur and Weiss 2009). The suggestion that more attention be paid to the relationship among pandemics, health systems, societal and economic insecurity, and political violence was politically and institutionally welcome among the UN membership at that time. It was also linked to two of the most significant political agendas of the moment: human security and sustainable development (UNDP 1994).

From 1995 to 2003, the process of drafting the revised regulation continued, but there was concern that the initiative lacked the drive and diplomatic will to see its completion (Davies, Kamradt-Scott, and Rushton 2015: chap. 1). Annual reports to the WHA discussed pilot studies of syndromic surveillance and occasional regional consultation meetings on the pilot study findings, but it was a new infectious disease—SARS—that would be crucial in delivering the diplomatic momentum that had been lacking. In the space of two years, states agreed upon an expanded and revised IHR.

The first human infections of a zoonotic respiratory illness, SARS, originated in China in late 2002; and, by February 2003, Canada, Hong Kong, Viet Nam, and Singapore were reporting suspected caseloads of a respiratory illness of unknown origin. In a situation where there was no instrument available to direct and coordinate the response, the WHO Communicable Disease Cluster in Geneva, led by Dr. David Heymann and overseen by the WHO director-general, Dr. Gro Harlem Brundtland, quickly adapted. Facilitating the co-operation and coordination with the WHO Western Pacific—which had the membership of states most affected—the virus was sequenced and identified by 27 March 2003. In the meantime, the WHO director-general referred to the IHR when releasing travel advisories on countries and issued two travel advisories against China and Canada. Advice against travel to China was released twice by the WHO director-general in an effort to compel the country to cooperate with reporting its suspected caseload of SARS cases—which it eventually did (Cortell and Peterson 2006). By July 2003, the worst of the outbreak was thought to be over. During this time, the actions of the WHO had illustrated the capability of a robust IHR that—if applied in the way it was to SARS—could be flexible in responding to cooperative as well as recalcitrant states to secure prompt alerts and containment at the source (Heymann and Rodier 2004).

In May 2003, the annual WHA was being held in Geneva while the SARS outbreak was still unfolding. China was only just starting to release figures that detailed the true extent of the spread of the disease in Beijing and Guangzhou (two cities most affected). At the Fifty-Sixth WHA (Resolution 56.29) it was unanimously agreed to fast-track the IHR revisions and to meet in 2005 to adopt the revised instrument. The fear in 2003 was threefold—that the pace of SARS's spread could see the virus evolve and become more infectious, states could become reluctant to report an outbreak for fear of its effect on the passage of travel and trade, and poorly resourced health systems might have cases but not know because of an incapacity to detect and trace the outbreak. These concerns dominated the drafting negotiations in 2003 and 2004. Regional consultations with member states, led by the WHO and its regional offices, focused on several critical questions: What detection and response capacities should the revised IHR demand of states? What detection and response capacities should be demanded of the WHO? And what events should be the concern of a revised IHR? (Davies, Kamradt-Scott, and Rushton 2015: chap. 2). While the dominant concern in 2003 and 2004 was the spread and mutation of SARS, older priorities were also resurfacing, such as bioweapon attacks (in light of the anthrax letter attacks in the United States in late 2001). A year of regional consultations followed, and in May 2005, after days of contentious diplomatic discussions in Geneva, the draft instrument was passed as Resolution 58.3 the World Health Assembly on 23 May 2005.

Ten years later, it has been argued that there is no doubt SARS inspired the diplomatic will necessary to see the revised instrument passed (Heymann and West 2014). The IHR adopted in 2005 were unprecedented in both scope and specificity (Baker and Fidler 2006; Mack 2006; Whelan 2008; Hardiman

From IHR (1969) to IHR (2005): a major paradigm shift

- From control at borders to [also] *containment at source*
- From a list of diseases to *all public health threats*
- From preset measures to *adapted response* (WHO 2007b: 65)

2012). Now it was a matter of implementing what states had agreed to in the revisions.

The shift of the 2005 IHR instrument from its 1969 version is shown as a graph that the WHO often provided in PowerPoint presentations and publications on information concerning the new IHR (WHO 2007a: 11; see box).

Briefly below, I present how the revised IHR represented a paradigm shift for both the WHO and states from the prior instrument in three ways.

Containment at the Source

In Article 2 of WHA58.3, all member states of the WHA agreed that the scope and purpose of the instrument was "to prevent, protect against, control and provide a public health response to the international spread of disease in ways that are commensurate with and restricted to public health risks" (WHO 2008: Article 2). In adopting this legal framework, states agreed that they would share with the WHO (which includes the WHO headquarters in Geneva, the WHO country office within their country [if applicable], and the relevant WHO regional office) their suspicion of a potential Public Health Emergency of International Concern, "irrespective of origin or source" within 24 hours, and this obligation to report extends beyond a state's own territory. A PHEIC was defined as

an extraordinary event which is determined, as provided in the Regulations:

(i) to constitute a public health risk to other States through the international spread of disease and

(ii) to potentially require a coordinated international response. (WHA 2005: 8)

Article 2 required states to not only report outbreaks but to "prevent, protect against, control" an outbreak *at the source*. The revised IHR included multiple references to states having the "capacity" to facilitate the detection of an outbreak at the local level, and the response and verification at the national level, and then capacity to contain or, failing this, to notify neighboring states and the WHO of the event (see WHO 2008: Articles 5, 13, 19, 20. 21, 44). With the exception of the Framework Convention on Tobacco Control (adopted in 2003), the revised IHR placed expectations on member states and the WHO that were unprecedented. Member states were being asked to agree to a revised IHR that demanded states to build core capacities in their public health system across eight areas: (1) national legislation, (2) policy and financing, (3) coordination and National Focal Point (NFP) communications, (4) surveillance and response, (5) preparedness, (6) risk communication, (7) human resources, and (8) laboratories (WHO 2008; for discussion, see Fischer and Katz 2013: 153–156). These became known as the IHR core capacities.

"Containment at the source" was not just an expansion of what the WHO could report but an expansion of what states could expect and demand from each other in the first instance of an outbreak event (Elbe 2010). This shift toward states having a responsibility to contain—not just report—disease outbreaks was discussed among regions in the drafting sessions in 2004. It did not go unnoticed at the time that meeting the functions listed under the eight core capacities, listed in full as Annex 1 attached to the IHR (2005), placed a significant demand on states with poor public health system capacity. Were states being "set up" to fail? There was a risk that the revised IHR were in many respects a continuation of the prior IHR, where states with capacity could respond to and manage an outbreak, while those without capacity would be "blamed" for outbreaks or continue to attach more value to hiding outbreaks than reporting their existence.

Before and during the 2005 WHA discussion (Whelan 2008), it was acknowledged that not all member states would achieve the eight core capacities by the time frame set—1 July 2012—and therefore two "sweeteners" were introduced to facilitate the adoption of the IHR with their core capacity requirements (Fidler 2005). First, a grace period was included in the revised instrument—three additional years could be requested to meet the IHR core capacity requirements. Under the IHR reporting mechanisms, states were expected to notify the WHO director-general of the need for an extension and identify the capacities where they still required assistance to achieve the benchmarks by 2015 (at the latest). However, the grace period would not be a private exchange between the WHO director-general and the state. From 2012, the WHO director-general was expected to provide an annual report to the WHA detailing which states had met their core capacity requirements and which had not. This was to be a very public forum. It was therefore expected, when the IHR was signed, that this public reporting process would accelerate states' commitment to the meet the IHR core capacities (Rodier 2007). The public naming and shaming exercise would benefit those states that had "made the grade" and, it was claimed, compel those falling behind to catch up.

The second sweetener was the suggestion of a funding mechanism to facilitate the adoption of the core capacity requirements requested by low- and middle-income countries during the draft IHR revision process. This led to the inclusion in the revised IHR of the suggestion in Article 44 that the WHO would mobilize "financial resources to support developing countries in building, strengthening and maintaining the capacities provided for in the Appendix (Core Capacities for Surveillance and Response)" (WHO 2008: Article 44 [2.c]).

The delay and the financial inclusion smoothed the path for additional inclusions in the revised IHR: the requirement that states communicate to the WHO within 24 hours of outbreak detection and within 48 hours to confirm the event, the WHO's right to receive reports of suspected outbreaks from non-state actors, and self-reporting surveys on individual state progress in meeting the eight core capacities that would be presented to the WHA by the WHO director-general from 2012 (five years after the instrument came into force). These measures were adopted without opposition in the 2005 WHA and gave the WHO the tools to demand better performance from states in disease outbreak surveillance and detection (Heymann and West 2014). Securing support for these revisions was essential to secure consensus that prevention and containment at the source was each state's responsibility as a signatory to the IHR. What remained unknown was whether this instrument could serve as the opportunity to address the long-standing public health capacity gap among countries while also addressing states' heightened sense of biosecurity vulnerability.

All Public Health Threats

The revised IHR awarded the WHO director-general a more proactive role in obtaining reports of outbreak events from states within a 48-hour time frame. The new focus was on ensuring timely containment measures and advice at the source of the public health emergency. This was in contrast to the prior method of states notifying the WHO (with no time frame specified) of an outbreak and then the WHO advising on the containment measures to be implemented in the affected and neighboring states at the ports of entry (air, sea, and land). Under the new arrangements, the WHO was to be notified of an outbreak within a specific time frame, could recommend steps to *contain* the outbreak, and, failing that, could formally *notify* the international community. The WHO was even permitted to act upon reports of outbreak events from sources *other* than the state and was granted a right to keep the identity of the informant confidential, ostensibly to protect that informant from repercussions by the state (see Baker and Fidler 2006). The definition of a public health event was expanded beyond a specific list of diseases (former IHR) to a matrix system that permitted the WHO director-general, in consultation with a specially convened IHR Emergency Committee, to prepare advice and guidance on a range of "all public health" events that could constitute a potential Public Health Emergency of International Concern (Annex 2, WHO 2008).

The revised IHR significantly broadened the concept of public health risk—the diseases and events that could trigger international action—and the WHO's authority to respond and provide advice in these circumstances. First, consistent with the 1948 WHO Constitution, disease was broadly defined as "an illness of medical condition, irrespective of origin or source, that presents or could present significant harm to humans." Second, a potential PHEIC "event" required the WHO to communicate with the affected state about the situation if it signified "a manifestation of disease or an *occurrence* that creates a potential for disease" (emphasis added). Finally, a "public health risk" could be declared and require WHO intervention (to assist and advise affected states and the broader international community), when the "likelihood of an event that may affect adversely the health of human populations, with an emphasis on one which may spread internationally or may present a serious or direct danger" (WHO 2008: Article 1d). Additionally, the revised IHR permitted the WHO director-general to declare a PHEIC without the "permission" of the affected state—the director-general may hear the concerns of the affected state, but it would be the director-general's decision to convene an Emergency Committee to discuss the event, to declare the PHEIC (after consultation with the IHR Emergency Committee, which includes representatives from the country originally infected), and to terminate the PHEIC (Articles 48 and 49).

A public health emergency of international concern requires states to identify and report public health risks—even those outside their territory—if they may pose an international threat (WHO 2008: Articles 6, 7, 9 and 11). This requires the WHO, at the regional or headquarters level, to engage in a process of verification with the affected state. Depending on the extent of the outbreak, the type of outbreak, and the cooperation of the state involved, the WHO director-general may then convene an IHR Emergency Committee (as noted above, a new committee is convened for each event) to "make temporary recommendations in order to prevent or deduce the international spread of disease and to minimize interference with international traffic." WHO director-general

Dr. Margaret Chan convened the first IHR Emergency Committee in 2009 in response to H1N1 influenza outbreak; she convened five more Emergency Committees up to the end of her tenure in 2017. Seven Emergency Committees have been convened and four PHEICs have been declared since the IHR came into force: the H1N1 Emergency Committee in 2009 (which declared H1N1 as a PHEIC), the MERS Coronavirus Emergency Committee in 2013 (no declaration), the Wild Poliovirus Emergency Committee in 2013 (a PHEIC declaration), the Ebola Emergency Committee in 2014 (a PHEIC declaration), the Zika Emergency Committee in 2016 (a PHEIC declaration), the Yellow Fever Emergency Committee in 2016 (no declaration), and the 2018 IHR Emergency Committee for Ebola virus disease (no declaration yet). The H5N1 avian influenza outbreak (peak phase between 2004 and 2009 in Southeast Asia and Egypt) never led to the convening of an IHR Emergency Committee. The suspect human-to-human transmissions occurred between the adoption of the IHR in 2005 and prior to the IHR coming into force in 2007. However, at the peak of the outbreak in poultry- and animal-to-human transmission in 2006, the WHA adopted Resolution 59.2, which declared that the international community should respond to the outbreak as if the revised IHR were already in force (WHA 2006).

In 2007, when the IHR came into force, the WHO argued that this instrument would be engaged with epidemic-prone diseases but also food-borne diseases, accidental and deliberate biochemical outbreaks, toxic chemical incidents, radioactive accidents, and environmental disasters (Rodier 2007). Most observers had little expectation that PHEICs would be regularly announced, but it was expected that there would be the normalization of the WHO's engagement in providing technical advice to states and convening committees to discuss and advise on situations to overcome the prior stigma of states seeking international assistance to deal with outbreak events (Ijaz et al. 2012). Some went so far as to suggest that the revised IHR could normalize the regular creation of IHR Emergency Committees to deal with outbreak events and the engagement of the WHO director-general in local outbreaks and disasters that required technical advice (Fidler and Gostin 2008: 149–150). Indeed, Kohl and colleagues point to the normalization of exchanging health information as the added value of the revised IHR—notifications become easier when they are done often (Kohl et al. 2014). To facilitate the normalization of reporting, it has even been suggested that there be a rotating Emergency Committee for a specified term, rather than a creating a new committee for each outbreak (Gostin and Katz 2016). Travel and trade would be less affected, it was hoped, if IHR Emergency Committees became the norm rather than the exception. In turn, states would be less fearful of travel and trade repercussions and engage in transparent reporting when required. The regularization of convening IHR Emergency Committees was not the practice of Chan, the WHO director-general with the longest record of presiding over the revised IHR. This means that the very convening of an IHR Emergency Committee has become a significant—and potentially controversial—political move, since it opens the door to the potential triggering of measures that could impact negatively on a country's trade and travel arrangements (a crucial factor in the early days of the Ebola outbreak in 2014). It remains to be seen whether her successor, Dr. Tedros Adhanom Ghebreyesus, will alter this course and normalize the convening of IHR Emergency Committees.

Adapted Response

Since the IHR came into force in 2007, signatory states have been expected to meet their core capacity requirements under the new framework.[5] Within the IHR, member states committed themselves to build core capacities in the areas of national legislation, policy and financing, coordination and NFP communications, surveillance, response, preparedness, risk communication, and human resources and laboratories (WHO 2008: Articles 5, 13, 19, 43). It was presumed at the outset that not all member states would achieve these eight capacities by the time frame set—1 July 2012—and the regulations included a clause to permit further extension of two years (Articles 5, 50). By the end of 2013, 118 member states (of 194 states) had requested an additional two-year extension to build requisite core capacities (WHO 2014: 6).

Multiple extensions were built into the IHR framework because the revised framework demanded more resource commitment from member states, both in prevention and containment. The evident difficulties for these 118 states in meeting the IHR core capacities are largely rooted in general health system deficiencies—not all health systems are equal—not to mention differentiated disease burdens that require time and investment in addition to meeting IHR core capacity requirements (WHO 2014: 9). This fact was originally acknowledged in the revised IHR with the expectation that there would be additional investment to assist developing states build the eight capacities, particularly surveillance and response, to meet the core functions of the IHR (WHO 2008: Article 44).

As noted above, the expectation that the WHO would be more proactive in presiding over an expanded IHR was tempered by the confidentiality conditions attached to the reporting practice of the revised IHR. One trade-off for the expanded definition of a public health threat was the transition from an open outbreak notification list published weekly to a private member state–only notification and a verification list managed by the WHO (MacKenzie and Merianos 2013). A state-appointed IHR National Focal Point (the post may rotate among designated individuals) is responsible for being available on a 24-hour, seven-day-a-week basis to respond to WHO requests for information, and the focal point has access to a WHO-administered event management system. Outbreaks are still reported (but subject to time delay) on an open list—*Disease Outbreak News* (*DON*)—but the WHO-administered event management system can receive notification and report notices that are immediate and focal point subscriber–only. As noted above, this server was created in exchange for the expanded reporting powers of the IHR. Of course, this system of reporting under the IHR makes it difficult to independently verify and track the degree to which states are complying with the "report early and often" expectation of the revised IHR (Rodier 2007). Unsurprisingly, the international community primarily hears about the events where notification was delayed (with some exceptions; see Liverani and Coker 2012). These reports inevitably lead to public discussion about the effectiveness of WHO and low-capacity states in responding to disease outbreaks (see Gostin and Friedman 2015; Moon et al. 2015). The degree to which this concern is an accurate measure of the problem remains unknown. The nature of confidential reporting is that the event management system rarely publicizes its success. What we do know is that the expanded reporting purview was adopted and that this development was novel—for WHO and its member states—and not entirely uncontentious (MacKenzie and Merianos 2013). Below, I will introduce the narratives that surround the IHR implementation record to date and the current status of IHR implementation region by region, and then, in the rest of the book, I will examine the specific case of IHR implementation in the Southeast Asia region.

The IHR since 2007: Three Narratives

In first six months of 2014 the WHO secretariat chose not to convene an IHR Emergency Committee to discuss the first recorded outbreak of Ebola hemorrhagic fever across three West African states as it spread from the index case in Guinea (December 2013 outbreak confirmed in March 2014) to Liberia (March 2014) and Sierra Leone (March 2014). It was not until its spread into Nigeria (June 2014) and the first suspected infection of a US citizen that the WHO director-general convened the Emergency Committee

(July 2014) and declared a PHEIC under the terms of the IHR on 8 August 2014.

The outbreak caused more than 20,000 deaths in West Africa, primarily in Guinea, Liberia, and Sierra Leone. It took well over a year to bring the infection under control in these three countries, and fear remains high that an outbreak will return to a region that had never experienced an Ebola outbreak prior to 2014. Outbreaks of deadly violence occurred in Liberia and Guinea, and emergency rule was introduced in both countries (S. Davies 2017). Medical workers were threatened with arrest if they failed to turn up to work or if they reported information that contradicted their government in all three countries. Risk communication messages were often uncoordinated and distrusted by the local populations. Mass displacement of populations from cities and affected villages occurred—people fled in fear for their lives or in a desperate search for sparse opportunities for medical care—and this movement made it difficult to trace cases and detect the extent of the outbreak.[6] The UN Security Council approved its first-ever mission in response to an infectious disease outbreak, the UN Mission for Ebola Emergency Response in September 2014. Coordination was shared between the UN Office for Coordination of Humanitarian Affairs and the WHO, but the first head of the Ebola response was not a WHO official but a UN secretary-general-appointed special representative, Anthony Banbury, who was assistant secretary-general for field support (UN Department of Peacekeeping). This was an unmistakable message that the WHO was no longer in charge of the international response to an outbreak that it had the purview to contain under the 2005 IHR. The media reported this as a monumental failure on the behalf of the WHO, and a thousand articles bloomed examining where the WHO had gone wrong (Fidler 2015; Gronke 2015; McInnes 2015; Moon et al. 2015; Paxton 2015; Sengupta 2015; Kamradt-Scott 2016).

In addition to the debate about the WHO's response were questions about the efficacy of the IHR revisions in shaping state behavior in response to public health emergencies. The devastation caused by Ebola was no doubt heightened by the fact that the outbreak occurred in three countries with some of the worst health indicators and systems. Sub-Saharan Africa accounts for 24% of the world's disease burden—populations requiring medical assistance and care on a regular basis—but the population has access to only 3% of the total health care workers available worldwide (WHO 2006: 8). And this trend has worsened since 2006 (WHO 2016c: 45). All three of the worst-affected countries—Guinea, Liberia, and Sierra Leone—were postconflict countries receiving financing from the UN Peacebuilding Fund. At the time of the outbreak, a UN peacekeeping mission was still deployed in Liberia. Likewise, Guinea too was on the agenda of the UN Security Council owing to protracted political instability, a series of coups, and electoral violence. Guinea and Sierra Leone's under-five mortality rates are 11th and 5th highest among the 54 countries in the African Union (African Health Stats 2016a). Sierra Leone, followed by Liberia, held 1st and 7th place for highest maternal mortality (Guinea is 11th for this indicator) (African Health Stats 2016b).

Health system reform in postconflict countries had been deemed "essential"—as the 2007 WHO report had outlined—for the IHR to deliver a "safer world" (WHO 2007b). Guinea had never reported on its status of compliance to the IHR core capacities, while Liberia and Sierra Leone had last reported their status in 2011 and both reported a low status of progress across the eight capacities. Simply put, there is no evidence that the IHR were a priority for any of these three states. By 2014, it had undoubtedly become a priority; Ebola had a devastating impact on the health of women and children, which was *already* substandard in these countries. Pervasively weak health systems were struggling to contain an outbreak where not one of the countries most affected had more than one physician available for every 1,000 persons. The general consensus was that the process for notification, verification, and response under the IHR had failed in these countries, the WHO had failed to connect fragile political systems to the transparent reporting processes, and the WHO had failed to raise the alert in making the connection between poor health system capacity and outbreak effective response.[7]

The Ebola outbreak in West Africa was seen as a symptom of the limitations of the revised IHR on disease outbreak response and containment attributable to three constraints within the WHO as an institution and in its relationship to states. First, the IHR permitted the continuation of the WHO's dysfunctional, decentralized structure (Sridhar and Gostin 2011; Youde in Gronke 2015). Under the revised IHR, states could continue to avoid reporting to the headquarters and direct their notifications to the WHO regional office. The implication here, as it was in the case of the Ebola outbreak, is that regional organizations may be more politically sensitive to the concerns of member states. There is dissention here. Some in AFRO (the WHO's Regional Office for Africa) have argued they did make it clear that countries were not coping, while others point to AFRO as repeatedly asking WHO headquarters to engage discreetly with affected countries (Boseley 2015; Sengupta 2015). This was a pattern that had been commonly adopted by the WHO and countries. As Kamradt-Scott (2016) points out, the WHO response in 2014 was in convention with previous Ebola outbreaks, if not greater. The WHO mobilized more than 100 staff through the Global Outbreak Alert Response Network (GOARN) in April 2014 when the outbreak in Guinea was confirmed as Ebola in late March. Discreet messages are often conveyed from the regional organization to headquarters—sometimes even bypassing the members-only event management system. This pattern of reporting was adopted because outbreak messages may convey points of political sensitivity. Done discreetly, they can be delivered without "raising the alarm" and in a way that ensured an ongoing reporting relationship with the affected state. It was precisely this arrangement in the case of Guinea (the first affected state) and AFRO that led to, it has been argued, WHO headquarters failing to respond to the speed and gravity of the Ebola outbreak. It is thought that removing or diminishing the role of the "third wheel"—the regional office—and normalizing reporting directly from the state to headquarters provides an opportunity to institutionalize the regular function of state reporting to headquarters. Indeed, since the Fifty-Ninth WHA (2016), this has become the proposed reporting structure for future outbreak events approved by the WHA—with WHO country offices to report directly to WHO headquarters (WHA 2016b).

The second critique of the IHR relates to the instrument itself. The IHR are a comparatively weak international instrument with no external review process for state compliance. Arguably, this permits states to take it less seriously compared to other instruments that have periodic reporting requirements (Giorgetti 2012: 1374). Compare, for example, the reporting requirements to international human rights instruments that fall under mandate of the UN Human Rights Council—whose state performance comes under Universal Periodic Review (UPR) every five years. In addition to the UPR, compliance with individual treaties (to which they are signatories) periodically come under review by human rights treaty bodies attached to each treaty (there are more than 10 treaty bodies). Civil society groups are entitled to contribute to these processes and provide shadow reports on states' performance. The Office of the High Commissioner on Human Rights also reports periodically on compliance with international human rights law. There is no similar formal opportunity for civil society to engage in the IHR process at the WHA or anywhere else in the WHO structure (Gostin and Katz 2016). Nor is the WHO secretariat entitled to conduct independent evaluations and report on individual states.

Why is this opportunity for multi-stakeholder review important? It is sometimes alleged that the IHR's reporting mechanisms are overdependent on self-reporting by states and that there is no alternative shadow reporting or oversight by the WHO or civil society. The positive value of such mechanisms found in the Human Rights Council is that states accrue and seek legitimacy from being seen as compliant, states are generally reluctant to voice their opposition to fulfilling these rights, and these reporting rituals permit civil society to capture states' rhetoric to demand reform. Meanwhile, consensus is often forged from these processes to refine and extend non-derogative human rights (Kalin 2015: 33). The IHR's annual self-reporting mechanism gives states an implicit right to opt in, something reinforced by the fact that there are no repercussions for states that choose not to report to the WHO director-general on their core capacity progress or that offer misleading reports. This problem was identified relatively early. In 2011, the *Review of the Review Committee on the Functioning of the International Health Regulations (2005) in relation to Pandemic (H1N1) 2009* noted that the real concern was that a large number of states were not going to meet the 2012 core capacities deadline and it was not clear to these states that there would be any implications for failing to do so (WHA 2011: 13).

Finally, some critiques focus on the IHR implementation process. While training and workshops have been prioritized from the moment the IHR came into force, it has been largely up to states individually to secure the investment needed to achieve the IHR core capacities. Some of the capacities—such as the assignment of NFP, risk communication strategy, reforming legislation and policy to meet IHR reporting and port of entry requirements—do not require large expenditures. Nor could expenditures be directed toward equipping all 190-odd countries with sophisticated laboratories and surveillance systems, while human resourcing public health staff requires training and time, as well as money. But even the "low-cost" capacities require changes in behavior, reorganization of priorities, and political support over a substantial period. The fact is that the world's wealthier states opted against establishing a mechanism to boost investment in building capacity to support IHR implementation: this reduced the incentives and the increased the costs of compliance for states with significant capacity shortfalls (Aldis 2008; Calain and Sa'Da 2015).

In the case of the Southeast Asian states that I examine in the remainder of this book, we see that these concerns about the IHR are applicable to this region to a point. The self-reporting mechanism under the IHR was a point of contention in the development of the APSED framework (see chap. 4). States from the SEARO and WPRO regional offices have had a fair degree of autonomy in deciding when to participate in external evaluations of their IHR compliance, which has led to differentiation in how states judge their IHR readiness. I argue that what has tempered the inclination to conduct glowing accounts of individual self-assessment has been the continued epistemic and political regional engagement in what IHR readiness looks like in action. This is, I contend, the normative influence of a regional framework pertaining to the IHR.

As such, even those states keen to present themselves as IHR ready in the early years (e.g., Cambodia and Myanmar) have come to temper their self-assessment of IHR readiness in the later years. Meanwhile, states such as Indonesia, Laos, and Viet Nam have always approached the IHR self-assessment exercise with a fair degree of honesty within the region. Participating in regional evaluation exercises and regional workshops in the first phase of implementation (2005–2010) was, I show, vital for sharing IHR implementation stories. By 2010 this region already demonstrated stronger IHR compliance in detection and reporting performance (Chan et al. 2010). The more troubling aspect of the IHR in the regional context, and this is particularly clear in the Southeast Asian region, is the degree to which compliance and readiness depend almost entirely on state-led (and state-controlled) engagement. This is a point I return to and discuss more fully in chapters 5 and 6.

IHR in Perspective

A more global perspective on the IHR, one that includes signs of progress as well as failure, would suggest that—contrary to the positions described above—some progress, albeit uneven, has still been made. Since the Ebola outbreak in West Africa, there have been two WHO-appointed reviews of the institutional response to the Ebola outbreak, one UN Secretary-General High Level Panel on the Global Response to Health Crises, and four high-profile specially convened international commissions (from civil society, academia, and policy) to investigate the IHR core capacity performance among states, the prioritization of WHO reform, and the structure of global health governance to support IHR implementation and WHO reform (Gostin et al. 2016). A consistent message across these reviews has been that IHR core capacity compliance is failing. Often the following statistic is provided: two-thirds of 193 UN member states are not fully compliant with the eight core capacities under the IHR. In real numbers, the argument is that five years since the 2012 deadline, 128 states have not met the eight core capacities. Of these 128 states, "only" 118 requested a two-year extension until 2014 to meet their capacity targets (which was granted).

The UN secretary-general appointed a High Level Panel on the Global Response to Health Crises reported in 2016:

> At present, 65 States Parties (33 per cent) have indicated that they have met the minimum Core Capacity standards; 84 (43 per cent) have requested an additional two-year extension; and 44 (22 per cent) have not communicated their status to the WHO. In May 2015, the World Health Assembly (WHA) granted a further extension of two years for all countries having requested it, bringing the deadline for full IHR compliance to 2016. (High Level Panel 2016: 32)

The High Level Panel recommended that 2020 was now a more realistic time frame for the extension and gave time to ensure that necessary funding and political mechanisms are in place to support those lagging states (32).

Below I examine the compliance performance of 193 states across the eight core capacities, comparing the self-report surveys provided by states in 2010 (125 states) and 2015 (117 states).[8] I contend that the prevailing critical view of IHR compliance fails to accommodate two important trends. First, most states take reporting their status more seriously. This is not a "tick and flick" exercise. A majority of states are providing detailed reporting on their capacity and are attempting to progress their core capacity requirements. This is a positive outcome for an instrument that was not yet 10 years old in 2015 (the instrument came into force in 2007). Significantly, states were doing this in the absence of any financial mechanism to support additional investment.

Second, while there are some interesting regional differences, the overall trend, from the worst-performing region (African regional office member states) to the best-performing region (Western Pacific regional office member states), was positive. Across the board, states are getting closer—not further away—from achieving the core capacity goals. Given this, it seems unlikely that the observed shortfall in capacity stems from the legal weakness of the IHR, structural weakness of the WHO, or a lack of political will on the part of states. Viewed globally, the key point is that the great majority of states are reprioritizing their policies and health systems to achieve the core capacities. There is, I contend, a deeper story to be told here about the states that are taking the IHR seriously, and we are yet to discover their stories of self-reporting and compliance. This is the story the rest of the book will explore, specific to the Southeast Asian region. This narrative is vital to understand the economic, social, and political conditions in which a government decides share outbreak information with its neighbor. It is also vital to progress and assist the effort the majority of states have made to become IHR compliant.

Signs of Progress

States have reached different stages of progress toward meeting their IHR core capacity functions. There were 44 states that the WHO reported in 2016 as having never provided information on their progress toward the IHR, but this is out of 193 states that have reported (in some capacity) since 2010. If we look at a comparison of state performance between 2010 and 2015, we see a story of progress. Here I compare the progress of responses to IHR core capacities between 2010 and 2015. The range that states could self-report their progress was 0%–24%, 25%–49%, 50%–74%, and 75%–100% compliance. In 2010 193 countries were surveyed, 125 responded and 68 did not (NA). In 2015, 193 countries were again surveyed and 76 did not respond (NA), while 117 responded. The overall story between 2010 and 2015 across the eight core capacities is, as figures 1.1 and 1.2 show, progressive, though predictably uneven, compliance.

In 2010, 193 countries reported on their IHR core capacities progress (WHO 2017a); 68 countries reported no data on progress across the eight capacities. The most impressive shifts have been countries moving from the 50%–74% percent margin to the 75%–100% margin (from 2010 to 2015), and two capacities that dramatically changed from 0%–49% margins to the 50%–100% margins have been surveillance and human resource capacities. If we disaggregate IHR compliance by region (Africa, the Americas, the Eastern Mediterranean, Europe, Southeast Asia, the Western Pacific), the picture of revised IHR that are struggling, even failing, to influence state behavior is further undermined. There is no doubt that regions experience variation in their performance across the eight capacities. In fact, in the case of the Ebola outbreak, given the record of poor state-level IHR compliance in the African region (particularly from Guinea, Liberia, and Sierra Leone), the initial lack of activity from the WHO headquarters response is more vexing (Boseley 2015). However, what is remarkable is that, quite contrary to prevailing narratives, which suggest that the IHR have failed to promote compliance, the story between 2010 and 2015 is one of advancement across the eight capacities and the majority of states conducting reports are shifting toward the 50%–100% compliance standard. These shifts are occurring, crucially, among low- and middle-income countries across the five regions.[9]

Of course, the states whose progress cannot be accounted for are the ones that have not reported (and their status is a cause for concern: these countries trend second highest in figure 1.1 and figure 1.2).[10] The first thing to note is that a nonreporting state may have missed only that year, that is, 2010 or 2015, so

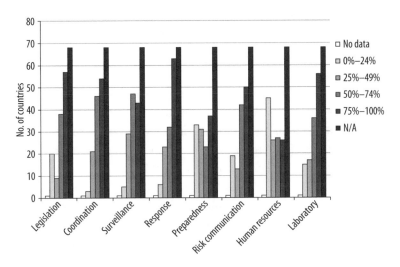

Figure 1.1. IHR Core Capacities, All Countries, 2010

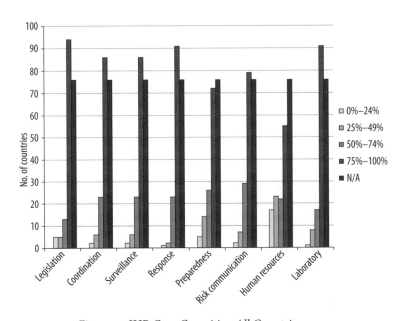

Figure 1.2. IHR Core Capacities, All Countries, 2015

these figures should be studied understanding the annual reporting requirement under the IHR. Thailand, for example, reported every year until 2015. The vast majority of Pacific Island states have reported once and then not again over the five-year time frame. The same may be said of a number of countries in the European region and Mediterranean region (e.g., Bulgaria, Iceland, Italy, Kyrgyzstan, Serbia, Turkey, Turkmenistan, the United Kingdom, Uzbekistan). Furthermore, the majority of countries that appear to make up the group of states that have never reported (the 44 group) are conflict and postconflict states primarily in sub-Saharan Africa (Somalia has reported since 2015, as have Côte d'Ivoire, Guinea, Guinea-Bissau, Liberia; no reports from Equatorial Guinea, Gabon, Madagascar, Senegal) and some small island countries part of the American regional office (Comoros, Haiti [reported once], St. Kitts, San Marino). Then there are states that have, again, reported once across the eight capacities or selectively reported for one or two capacities (e.g., Lesotho, Malawi, Mauritania, Nauru, Niue, Papua New Guinea, Rwanda, Zimbabwe).

In Core Capacity 1, which requires national legislative and budgetary reform, the legislation, policy, and financing reform measures (appendix: figure A.1) in 2010 were relatively strong. There were 95 countries reporting 50%–100% compliance in the three years since the IHR had come into force. By 2015, this number had risen to 114 countries, with the vast majority in the 75%–100% compliance zone. If we break this figure down by region (figure A.2) with the exception of the African region (29% compliance) and the American region (47%; PAHO), the other regions reporting their status were already more than halfway compliant: 67% for European region (EURO), 68% and 69% for South-East Asia and Eastern Mediterranean regions (respectively), and 71% for the Western Pacific (WHO 2017a). When assessed by region, as figure A.2 shows, Africa was the weakest performer in legislative reform to implement the IHR. However, by 2015 (and taking into account the Ebola outbreak in West Africa in 2014), the African region has tripled its compliance status for legislation reform, while the other regions were also showing strong progress with four out of five WHO regions reporting status in the 75%–100% zone.

A comparison of the regions from 2010 to 2015 in Core Capacity 2, National Focal Point, coordination and communication (figure A.3), also demonstrates the need to include or conduct a disaggregated study of the IHR compliance. If we look at the global trends from 2010 to 2015, the number of states achieving 75%–100% implementation has doubled. A large number of the countries rated in the 50%–74% category in 2010 have made that progressive shift to 75%–100% in 2015. The same shift is occurring between the 25%–49% status and 50%–74%

status. At the regional level (figure A.4), it may also be observed that all five regions have progressed in terms of overall compliance. The African region, again, is not performing strongly compared to the other regions, but it is making progress when compared to its own past practice. There are certainly no signs of stagnation across these first two vital core capacities—legislative reform and budget and financial reform, as well as the institutional reform necessary to coordinate the function of executive government in response to an outbreak. The pace is different from country to country and region to region, but so is the variation across political institutions, economic status, and health system capacity. A degree of unevenness is to be expected, given variations across countries and the intervention of exogenous events. The story of an IHR in crisis because less than a quarter of states (44 out of 193), many of them microstates, are not responding to the reporting expectation needs to be tempered. In addition, we need to remember that states with 100% compliance across the eight capacities, like Canada, Singapore, South Korea, and Saudi Arabia, can also face health emergencies that may challenge their public health systems (Gostin and Katz 2016).

Across the remaining six core capacities (figures A.5–A.16), the story is again one of general, but uneven, progress, with the vast majority of states moving toward the 50%–100% compliance bracket (two exceptions where progress has been slowest is human resourcing and preparedness). The slow positive growth in these two areas requires a brief discussion. In 2012, there were a number of publications on the need to refine evaluation and progress measurements of the revised IHR core capacities, as well as to ascertain the precise associated costs for implementation (Ijaz et al. 2012: 1054–1057; Katz et al. 2012: 1121–1127). Human resourcing—field-trained public health professionals and epidemiologists—was referred to in the Ijaz et al. article (2012: 1055) as "one of the first priorities of implementing the IHR"; and, in a study on the cost of full implementation of the eight IHR core capacities, Katz and colleagues (2012) estimated that for a Southeast Asian country with a population of 60 million, meeting the training requirements listed under the human resources capacity was one of the least-expensive core capacities to fund. Here we see a potential paradox where human resourcing should be a capacity that most states are progressing toward the 75%–100% group over the five years. Instead, it is the one capacity that has the lowest number of states meeting (60 states reported 75%–100% in 2015, up from 26 states in 2010; see figures A.13 and A.14).

Preparedness was not identified in the Ijaz et al. (2012) study as one of the four core capacities that can be easily monitored and evaluated for progress.

In the Katz et al. piece (2012), it becomes apparent why this is the case. Preparedness is both infrastructure and human resource intensive. It is also costly. Predictions are that US$100 million (per year) is needed just to stock surge capacity necessary to treat 100 patients and an upfront cost of US$2.8 million is required to build a climate-controlled stockpile storage facility. Then there is the need to fund annual salaries to manage the infrastructure as well as hire national emergency staff who are on call to respond to an event. Finally, there are costs involved in training and tabletop exercises for public health staff (who already have other jobs). This is where the human resource capacity shortfall starts to indicate why laboratory readiness, for example, may be adequate, but the picture of who will be doing the testing on the rotations needed to maintain flow of information and verification is less clear.

The Ijaz et al. (2012) study presented the argument that some indicators (human resourcing, surveillance, laboratory, and response) were more disposed to immediate measurement than others (legislation, policy, and financing; coordination; advocacy and NFP communications; preparedness; and risk communication). The cost for meeting the eight core capacities were, Katz et al. show (2012), potentially impossible for some countries, given their existing public health budgets and infrastructure, public health disease burden, and available public health staff. This prediction has proven correct and led to situations where states determine what capacities they can immediately meet, which will take more time, and which may never be suitable for them to devote resources and time to (Kool et al. 2012). As Katz et al. (2012: 1121) argue, the functional implementation of the IHR has required "flexibility for nations to determine how best to structure and develop these capacities."

As such, shortfalls in meeting preparedness capacity, for example, are understandable for a vast number of low- and middle-income countries that cannot justify such expenditures on large storage facilities for a particular outbreak that may or may not be suitable to that scenario (International Working Group on Financial Preparedness 2017: 64). Amid all the discussion on implementation of the IHR, human resources may be justifiably identified as an essential capacity and the one that needs the greatest attention and resource mobilization moving forward. It also has the potential to benefit communities during and outside of public health crises.

Disaggregation by capacity as well as by region therefore gives us the opportunity to study in more detail the trends for individual capacity shortfalls and regional capacity shortfalls, as I will show in the ASEAN case.

Understanding Compliance in the Case of the IHR

The obstacles to full implementation of the IHR have been well documented. At varying levels for both developing and developed states, the predicted obstacles were technical, resource, legal, and political (Baker and Fidler 2006). The revised IHR recognized that these obstacles would be present to some extent in *all* states, and those with weak health systems would need priority assistance rather than condemnation for failing to react during outbreak crises (Heymann and Rodier 2004; Rodier 2007). The 2007 WHO report *A Safer Future* devoted an entire chapter (WHO 2007b: chap. 5) to the importance of strengthening public health systems to secure populations from PHEICs and to meet the compliance standards of the IHR. It was equally stressed in the same report that strong public health systems would also remain vulnerable to cross-border outbreak events.

The WHO's purpose in 2007 was to construct a message of cooperation and solidarity. Meeting IHR core capacities would provide a strong foundation on which to detect and respond. The system's "real" vulnerabilities were not in the strength of states' laboratory capacities but in the collective willingness to share reports and cooperate during outbreak events (Baker and Fidler 2006; Heymann 2006). In other words, compliance reporting was promoted in 2007 as a story of progress, and reward was for effort rather than achievement. This message has been "flipped" to some extent over the succeeding decade in the external reviews of WHO and the revised IHR. Today, the narrative of compliance failure risks downplaying what has been achieved in a short time and the very real evidence that the IHR have exerted considerable "compliance pull" across a sizable majority of states.

The intention in 2005 was to mount a naming and shaming public relations exercise to encourage states to meet their individual implementation targets. Despite this measure, states have tended not to submit misleading reports claiming 100% compliance. The core capacity implementation deadline of 2015 was established to increase the pressure on states to devote resources and political will to the revised IHR (Rodier 2007). Despite the reporting variations across the core capacities shown above, it is clear that the majority of states across the regions are treating this annual exercise to self-report their status in a serious and reflective manner. Most states are not treating this exercise as a "tick the box" exercise and are seriously engaged with the process. As such, reporting capacity gains and capacity shortfalls should be rewarded rather than despaired.

Furthermore, looking at the bigger picture we see that a majority of states have moved toward greater compliance with the IHR. Yet, of course, there is much more to the story than this. We cannot understand how and when compliance has been achieved (or has failed) by looking only at aggregated tallies of which states have met all the IHR core capacities. A compliance score risks becoming the end in itself. However, before we presume what has worked and what has failed concerning IHR implementation to date, we need to identify whether there are regional experiences that challenge the overriding message that the revised IHR have been a political and technical failure. Are the functions and structures associated with the revised IHR—annual self-reporting, a decentralized WHO, and a legal instrument without coercive capacity—part of the problem or the source of the progress? Why have some states progressed more than others? Why have some capacities progressed more than others? Are there regional adaptions of the IHR that tell us the social and political story behind the technical aspects of IHR compliance?

At the macro/global level, it is difficult to ascertain precisely why states made the decisions that they did. All we can get is a macro-understanding that tells us that most states are complying more on most measures than they once did. A regional-level analysis provides one way of analyzing the local adaption of the revised IHR. At the regional level we may identify when and how states adopted particular stances, policies, or strategies and get a better understanding of the different priorities and concerns that confront decision makers with differentiated capacity to adapt. It is to the Southeast Asian case study that we now turn. The region stands out because of its immense health challenges, its commitment to principles of noninterference that would seem to directly contradict the IHR's reporting requirements, and its unique regional implementation program developed to pursue IHR compliance: the Asia Pacific Strategy for Emerging Diseases.

In the next chapter (chap. 2) I introduce the economic, political, social, and health background of the member states of ASEAN. Evaluating their political capacity is an important prelude to analyzing their fidelity to health security (chap. 3) and the principles of APSED and the IHR (chap. 4). The ASEAN states are particularly useful to study given that their membership spans both SEARO and WPRO, the two WHO regional offices that have collectively developed and promoted APSED.

Conclusion

The revised IHR were a response to the perceived shortcomings of existing international frameworks for responding to infectious disease risks. Until 2005, states decided what constituted a health threat to their citizens and responded accordingly; the WHO did not have authority to intervene or publicly suggest alternative recommendations (Fidler 2004a). Yet, under the revised IHR, the rules have changed. States can report public health concerns emanating from neighboring states, as can non-state actors; WHO can request information from states; states have to appoint a focal point to respond to these queries within a specified timeframe, which requires the surveillance and detection capacity to follow up these enquiries. Following all of this, the WHO director-general can then convene an IHR Emergency Committee to determine the nature of the threat and provide recommendations to the affected state (and the broader international community).

The IHR have deepened the surveillance and reporting expectations among states. A state can be judged on its capacity to respond to outbreak situations by its implementation status of the eight core capacities. The implementation reporting requirement was designed as a name and shame function that would compel states to meet the IHR core capacities, expose vulnerability and risk to neighboring states, and serve as a compliance pull. Variation, though inevitable, among 196 states in meeting the eight core capacities has undermined the rationalist argument that naming and shaming would alone compel states to act. Some states that are compliant no longer report, some that have never been compliant continue to fail to report, and some have treated the compliance exercise seriously and have been motivated to improve their implementation status, consistently reporting gradual improvement. The relationship among compliance, politics, economics, and regionalism has not been adequately understood to date.

There is significant variation in implementation across and within states (Katz et al. 2012; High Level Panel 2016). The remainder of this book explores the variation in the Southeast Asian experience to ask how—and why—a region committed to principles of noninterference not only accepted enhanced surveillance but has also taken steps to improve compliance with the IHR. This is a story of norm localization and adaption: how the region shaped its own shared sense of interests and pathways to implementation, prefaced on its own strategies and dense informal epistemic networks.

CHAPTER TWO

The Political Context in Southeast Asia

This chapter examines the political context in which the Southeast Asian government has confronted the management of infectious disease outbreaks. A diverse region, Southeast Asia houses democratic, partially democratic, and authoritarian states, many of which have experienced coups and other types of unconstitutional regime change and many of which had armed conflict in the past (e.g., Cambodia, Viet Nam, Indonesia), as well as some where armed conflict persists (e.g., Myanmar and the Philippines). In this context, it is perhaps not surprising that some of the region's states lack fully functioning health systems, supported by capable and stable institutions. This relationship among political regime type, health system capacity, and IHR core capacities is a vital yet considerably underexplored question. It is, I think, essential for understanding compliance (and noncompliance) with the IHR and is therefore the natural starting point for my investigation. We need to know precisely what is happening within a country if we are to understand and explain its level of compliance with the IHR. After all, some exogenous issues such as the political regime and presence of conflict could exert significant influence over national priorities that has nothing whatsoever to do with a government's views about the IHR themselves.

This chapter proceeds in three parts. First, I examine research on the relationship among health, political regime, political stability, and governance. Here I pay attention to the growing consensus that regime type matters insofar as it influences the capacity of states to build health systems that can promote the health of all. Second, I examine how this hypothesis sits with the Southeast Asian experience over a 20-year period—1990–2010 (the first year of IHR compliance reporting). The Southeast Asian case corroborates some of the key findings of the literature but challenges some other aspects—especially the relationship between democracy and health systems. The Southeast Asian case reveals that while democratic transition may deliver some political and social goods, it is not a necessary precondition for health system strengthening. However, political stability—the absence of conflict—is essential. This suggests states may not need to be democratic to do what is required to fulfill the IHR, but political stability certainly assists the IHR compliance project. Finally, I consider how this finding may illustrate the experiences of cooperation in the ASEAN environment in the specific area of disease outbreak surveillance and response.

Health Inequality and Governance

What is the relationship between a "healthy" public health system and governance? It is well established that the toll of worsened health care during armed conflict creates high economic and political burdens on already fragile post-conflict states (Plümper and Neumayer 2006; Justesen 2012; Urdal and Che 2013). This line of inquiry has led to further questions about the regime-related factors that cause some communities to be healthier than others and the effects of this on patterns of governance (Price-Smith 2002). Our understanding of the relationship among strong health systems, regime type, and political stability is largely informed by debates concerning the democratic peace thesis (Oneal and Russett 1997; Dafoe, Oneal, and Russett 2013; Schneider 2013) and the associated democratic welfare thesis. Simply put, these theses hold that democracies are more likely to be peaceful and to provide social welfare that is of benefit to the whole population than are nondemocratic regimes (Baum and Lake 2003; Mousseau, Hegre, and Oneal 2003; Grépin and Dionne 2013). Thus, existing studies in this area have explored the amplification of health inequalities due to conflict and war, the impact of political stability on the capacity of the regime to respond to health vulnerabilities, and the effect of regime type and public health expenditure on long-term prospects for baseline improvements in health (Ghobarah, Huth, and Russett 2004; Ruger 2005; Price-Smith 2009; Iqbal 2010). To date, however, the literature on IHR compliance has not attended much to these findings.[1] This section briefly looks at the underlying assumptions about democracy, political stability, and health system strengthening to understand the questions we should ask about political systems when evaluating IHR compliance by states.

Democracies tend to be more responsive to the needs and wishes of their citizens and less concerned about regime survival than are nondemocracies (Muntaner 2013; Mackenbach and McKee 2015; Patterson 2017). What is more, political stability and governance may be connected in complex ways. In *The Health of Nations*, Price-Smith theorized a "probabilistic relationship among diseases, state capacity, societal deprivation . . . that may assist to some extent in the prediction of state failure and intra-state violence in the future" (2002:

176). In *Contagion and Chaos*, he returned to this argument to describe how disease may function as a "stressor variable" that compromises the prosperity, legitimacy, structure cohesion, and security of sovereign states (Price-Smith 2009: 3). From this perspective, disease can contribute to the onset of conflict, and the practice of warfare itself can amplify disease contagion, increasing the burden of disease and further reducing the chances of sustainable peace (Ghobarah, Huth, and Russett, 2004).

International relations scholars and policy makers have become increasingly concerned with the insecurity created by health threats ranging from Ebola to bioweapons and, of late, the global economic burdens caused by rising rates of chronic disease in developed and developing states (McInnes and Lee 2006; Koblentz 2010; Gostin 2012). What the IR lens has introduced are different referent points—how health affects security (of the state), how security should be recalibrated to consider the (health) needs of individuals, and how health inequalities produce health insecurity for individuals and states (Elbe 2011). As articulated in the previous chapter, the presumption of the revised IHR is that reforms to public health systems to meet the IHR core capacities would arrest the conditions that give rise to health insecurity. The first point of departure in IR is to examine the nature of health insecurity. What is the relationship between weak health systems, political instability, and health inequalities? With specific reference to the revised IHR, can we expect all states with compromised governance capacities and health systems to meet the IHR core capacities without significant levels of external assistance?

Addressing health inequalities is integral to health and political stability more broadly (Patterson 2017). Fractured health systems and protracted health vulnerabilities within populations exacerbate their collective weaknesses (Iqbal 2010). This creates political tension in the prioritization of resourcing. Is IHR compliance the priority when infant mortality and maternal mortality are the highest disease burdens and the density of physicians is 1 per 10,000 population (the optimal ratio is 1 per 1,000)? Alternatively, the argument that the IHR core capacities require reforms from states that, in politically unstable situations, have other priorities may miss the point—creating any kind of functional health system capacity, even in the "narrow" area of infectious disease control, may have broader public health and political stability benefits (Kruk et al. 2015). Little research and policy engagement been done—to date—to establish whether political conditions prioritize IHR compliance.

From the available literature can we establish whether certain types of regimes are more likely to invest in public health programs such as the IHR? Of relevance to this study, is democracy or political stability a condition for cooperative health endeavors, such as effective cooperation at the state and regional level in disease outbreak surveillance and response? The consensus thus far seems to hold that, indeed, democracies are more likely to be politically stable than autocracies as well as more likely to allocate the public resources needed to address health inequalities (Lake and Baum 2001; Wigley and Akkoyunlu-Wigley 2011).

In addition to understanding the political conditions conducive to IHR compliance, studies have also pointed to how weak health systems place neighboring states at heightened risk and compromise their ability to cooperatively defend borders and populations from infectious disease outbreaks (Price-Smith 2009: 112–116).

Combined, these accounts make a series of significant claims regarding the relationship among health spending, regime type, and political stability that are of particular relevance to the IHR. First, health inequalities can give rise to political instability. This argument comes as no surprise to those who argue that the recent history of political instability in Guinea, for example, was a crucial factor in the initial spread of the Ebola virus between 2013 and 2014: the (compromised) practice of risk communication of the disease and public trust in the government's response to the disease (ICG 2015). Second, health inequalities are especially pronounced in the wake of armed conflicts, and these inequalities increase social discontent and foster instability. In the case of Liberia during the Ebola virus outbreak in 2014, the use of emergency powers heightened fears in slum areas of Monrovia that the government (up for reelection that year) was exaggerating the outbreak to ensure its reelection and redirect aid away from the population (Mulbah, Zondi, and Connolly 2015). Third, concerted financial and government efforts, including government investment of time and resources, can remedy health inequalities and, by implication, the risks associated with them. Government engagement, even if imperfect, is an automatic force for good in health system strengthening (Gevrek and Middleton 2016). Fourth, and crucial to the IHR project, democratic regimes seem more likely than nondemocratic regimes to make investments and positively engage in health system strengthening; correlated to this, they are less likely to experience political instability (which further enhances the population's health progress and health capacity building) (Klomp and de Haan 2009; Grépin and Dionne 2013; Mackenbach, Hu, and Looman 2013; Pega et al. 2013).

However, there are conditions that potentially affect the certainty of the relationship between regime type and positive health outcomes: namely, the length of time the country has been democratic and the contention that it is the quality of redistribution, not regime type, that determines health outcomes (Ross 2006). In the context of the revised IHR, how should these insights into political systems influence the compliance discussion? In the next section, I examine the relationship between political systems and health systems in Southeast Asia. This regional analysis is important for two reasons. First, it allows us to test the supposed correlation between IHR compliance and democratization in a non-Western context (Goldsmith 2013). Second, there are few regional-level analyses available that complement and further inform the global trends observed in the above literature (Iqbal 2010: 94).[2] As such, there have been few studies on whether this relationship remains evident in specific, regional contexts (see Perlo-Freeman 2012).[3]

The Southeast Asian[4] region is a mix of stable, postconflict, and low-intensity conflict states, with significant differences across regime type (Doner, Ritchie, and Slater, 2005; Kivimäki 2011; Goldsmith 2013). The remainder of this chapter examines the strength of the relationship between regime type and strengthening of the health system (represented as positive gains in lowering individual country disease burden and health expenditure) in Southeast Asia. An important caveat before we begin exploring the Southeast Asian case: I do not suggest that democracy is not a desirable end goal in and of itself. Instead, I am interested in whether political stability and democracy are necessary prerequisites for IHR core capacity and reporting compliance or whether those goals can be achieved in the absence of these conditions.

The Southeast Asian Experience

Since 1967 (the year ASEAN was formed with core members Indonesia, Malaysia, Philippines, Singapore, and Thailand) the majority of ASEAN member states have experienced some form of internal conflict (Cambodia, Indonesia, Malaysia, Myanmar, Philippines, Thailand, Viet Nam) or interstate war (Cambodia, Viet Nam, Laos). Only Brunei Darussalam and Singapore have avoided political destabilization of the kind experienced in the other states since the formation of ASEAN. Most ASEAN states have achieved the peaceful resolution of their internal conflicts. Of the two remaining conflicts, one is a low-intensity conflict in the Philippines, and, as of April 2014, the Bangsamoro Peace Process concerning the Mindanao archipelago has remained in place between the Philippine government and the Moro Islamic Liberation Front. The second is in Myanmar, where high levels of internal political violence continue despite the signing of a Nationwide Ceasefire Agreement in 2015 (which applies to more than half of the eighteen combatant groups across the state). Conversely, ASEAN has experienced a long peace and tolerance of differences in both political regime type and strategic outlook among the membership (Kivimäki 2011; Goldsmith 2013). This has been the purported success and paradox of the ASEAN regional organization in Southeast Asia (Dosch 2008).

The relative peace of states within the group is recent and born out of a particularly violent past. During the Cold War period (approximately 1945–1989), some of the most brutal mass-atrocity crimes and conflicts have occurred in Southeast Asia. Alex Bellamy (2014: 3–5) estimates that East Asia as a whole (including China, North and South Korea, and Japan) accounted for 50% of the world's cases of mass atrocities in the 1960s and 1970s. In Indonesia, for example, the 1965–1966 coup and putsch saw approximately 600,000 suspected communists and civilians massacred; from 1975 to 1998, approximately 90,000–200,000 civilians died as a result of Indonesian occupation of East Timor (now Timor Leste), and in the Acehnese conflict (1975–2005) at least 15,000 were reportedly killed. In Cambodia, the Khmer Rouge (1975–1979) were responsible for at least 1.5 million deaths (of a population of 8 million), and at least 500,000 civilians were killed by indiscriminate bombing by the United States during the Viet Nam War. In Viet Nam, at least 1.5 million civilians lost their lives during the 1961–1975 conflict. The civil war and US bombing campaigns led to at least 50,000 civilians losing their lives during the same period in Laos. After Viet Nam invaded Cambodia in 1979 to remove the Khmer Rouge, Cambodia was not declared postconflict until 1996, when it held its first elections. Myanmar has had ongoing ethnic conflicts and territorial disputes since independence in 1948 and has been under absolute military dictatorship from 1962 to 2011. The Myanmar population has endured the longest civil war and one of the longest terms of military dictatorship; the brutality of both have led to the death of the tens of thousands, displacement of hundreds of thousands inside the country and neighboring states, and the worst poverty indicators among the ASEAN group (ICG 2012). Although the overall number of armed conflicts in Southeast Asia has declined dramatically (Kivimäki 2012; Bellamy 2014), intrastate conflicts have continued as low-intensity conflicts (25 battle-related deaths or more, using Uppsala Conflict Data Program [UCDP] definitions) in the Philippines (Mindanao) and Thailand (Patani ethnic conflict in the south), and one high-intensity conflict within Myanmar (1,000 battle deaths or more, using UCDP definitions; UCDP 2017).

This history, and in particular the narrative concerning the region's dramatic 30-year transition from war to peace (Kivimäki 2011; Johnston 2012; Goldsmith

2013; Bellamy 2014), makes the Southeast Asian region a challenging health case study. In terms of health systems, Southeast Asian states have a diverse range of public and private health care models, as well as markedly different health burdens. For example, Brunei, Malaysia, Singapore, Thailand, and Viet Nam all have life expectancies above the world average, yet the average wages and personal expenditure on health care in Malaysia, Thailand, and Viet Nam is markedly below the annual incomes and personal health expenditure of individuals in Brunei and Singapore (Coker et al. 2011).

Importantly, in contrast to other regions with a violent past, Southeast Asia generates plenty of data. In 2012, the Institute for Health Metrics Evaluation (IHME), with the cooperation of the World Health Organization, updated the comprehensive Health-Adjusted Life Expectancy (HALE) measures and Disability-Adjusted Life Year (DALY) measures originally produced in 2000 and 2004, respectively. When the WHO first produced these measures, they were the first large datasets to measure and compare life expectancy across 191 countries taking into account disease burdens. The principle aim was to quantify the years lost by disease burden and type (DALY) and then to identify the life expectancy of populations using the HALE score, which summarizes years lived in less than ideal health and years lost from premature mortality to produce a single measure of average population health for an individual country. The IHME dataset, referred to as the Global Burden of Disease Study 2010, is the most comprehensive global health dataset available for tracing individual states' progress compared to their performance in the original DALY and HALE dataset (Salomon et al. 2012).

At the time of the revised IHR adoption and revision, the IHME DALY and HALE measures for 2010 are complete and available for all ASEAN member states (IHME 2013). Likewise, World Bank data is available for ASEAN member states' public health and military expenditure during this same period (World Bank 2017), while data from Polity IV and Uppsala Conflict Data Program is available for ASEAN states to measure regime type and conflict prevalence/intensity (see tables 2.1 and 2.2) (Marshall and Gurr 2014; UCDP 2017). Moreover, as the previous chapter noted, the Southeast Asian region has been consistent in reporting its IHR compliance data since 2010. This allows us to deepen the comparative analysis in health security literature by folding in the independent variables identified above as crucial for testing the relationship among political stability, public health and health expenditure, and regime type against IHR compliance. The relevant variables are (1) impact of conflict-postconflict environment (the presence of low-intensity conflict or civil unrest),

TABLE 2.1. 1990 Southeast Asian States: Status of Health Inequalities

1990	HALE 1990	HIV DALY*1990	Malaria DALY 1990	TB DALY 1990	Maternal Complications DALY 1990[1]	Polity IV 1990[2]	UCPD 1990[3]	Mil exp 1990 (%GDP)[4]	Health exp 1990 (%GDP)[5]
Brunei									
Cambodia	50.1	67	3	6	4	Neg88/War	Yes (high intensity)	2.1	1
Indonesia	56.2	166	8	2	6	Neg7	Yes (medium intensity)	0.9	0.52
Laos	48.3	157	7	5	4	Neg7	Yes (low intensity)	0	0.44
Malaysia	62.1	27	72	16	10	Pos4	No	2.4	1.3
Myanmar	48.6	134	3	4	7	Neg7	Yes (high intensity)	3.4	NA
Philippines	57.8	168	58	2	3	Pos8	Yes (medium intensity)	2.1	1
Singapore	66.4	45	159	30	21	Neg2	No	4.9	1.09
Thailand	63.2	19	35	13	6	Pos3	Yes (low intensity)	2.7	1
Viet Nam	59.5	166	22	5	3	Neg7	No	7.9	0.83

[1] HALE, HIV, Malaria, TB, and Maternal DALY 1990 (IHME 2013).
[2] Marshall and Gurr 2014.
[3] UCPD 2017.
[4] World Bank 2017: Military expenditure % of GDP (per country).
[5] World Bank 2017: Health expenditure % of GDP (per country).
*DALY score represents the disease burden ranking for that country in terms of years of life lost (YLLs) due to premature death from that disease (IHME 2013).

TABLE 2.2. 2010 Southeast Asian States: Status of Health Inequalities[*]

2010	HALE 2010	HIV DALY 2010	Malaria DALY 2010	TB DALY 2010	Maternal complications DALY 2010[1]	PolityIV 2010[2]	UPCD 2010[3]	Mil exp 2010 (%GDP)[4]	Health exp 2010 (%GDP)[5]
Brunei									
Cambodia	58	16	14	5	4	Pos2	No	1.6^	1
Indonesia	60.9	30	29	2	12	Pos8	No	0.7^	1*
Laos	55.9	45	20	7	6	Neg7	No	0.3*	1*
Malaysia	64.4	5	71	28	25	Pos6	No	1.6^	2*
Myanmar	55.6	4	6	2	14	Neg6	Yes (high intensity)	NA	NA
Philippines	60.3	113	76	3	5	Pos8	Yes (low intensity)	1.2^	1
Singapore	71.1	45	159	32	50	Neg2	No	3.7^	1^
Thailand	65.3	1	79	26	25	Pos4	Yes (low intensity)	1.5^	3*
Viet Nam	65.8	6	66	21	11	Neg7	No	2.5^	3*

[1] HALE, HIV, Malaria, TB, and Maternal DALY 1990 (IHME 2013).
[2] Marshall and Gurr 2014.
[3] UCPD 2017.
[4] World Bank 2017: Military expenditure % of GDP (per country).
[5] World Bank 2017: Health expenditure % of GDP (per country).
*Shading indicates the postconflict countries since 1990.

(2) disease burden (HALE and DALY infectious disease and maternal mortality ranking), (3) level of public health expenditure (comparative to military expenditure), and (4) regime type (Price-Smith 2002; Ghobarah, Huth, and Russett 2004; Iqbal 2010). A snapshot of the region in 1990 and 2010 (tables 2.1 and 2.2) shows trends for each state in the region.

What is observed here are basic changes between 1990 and 2010 in public expenditure, health outcomes, regime type, and political stability among 10 ASEAN member states. Prior to the adoption of the IHR and during the first five years of revised IHR reform, this region has responded to IHR reform coupled with existing health burdens, political transformation and competing budget priorities, as the following chapters discuss. This observation across two decades produces four findings about how we understand the relevant relationship among regime type, political stability, and health outcomes in a region-specific case. At the end of this section, I will analyze these four trends against the first year of IHR compliance reporting among the states.

First, concerning the argument that democratic regimes are more inclined to redistribution and thus we can expect IHR reform to progress more easily in democracies, the Southeast Asian region experienced a general drift toward increased provision for health and social welfare as a percentage of GDP; and this occurred irrespective of regime type. With the exception of Myanmar, where data were not available, the remaining states reduced their public expenditure on military equipment as a percentage of GDP. Some reductions were quite small—Indonesia, a democracy, has reduced its proportion from 0.9% (1990) to 0.7% (2010). Other countries have had notable reductions—Viet Nam, measured as an autocracy in both 1990 and 2010, had the largest reduction, from 7.9% (1990) to 2.5% (2010). Of course, in most cases, an increased GDP means that although the proportion spent on the military has declined, real spending on the military has increased, but the same rule will apply to public health spending (see below). Given that I am primarily interested in the relative allocation of resources to public health compared to other sectors of the government, this change in allocation for most ASEAN states, democratic or not, is significant.

The reduction in relative spending on defense occurred at the same time as significant increases in health expenditure as a proportion of GDP across all the region's states from 1990 to 2010. Singapore was the only exception, with decreased spending—which was nevertheless significantly higher than for other states. Generally speaking, public health expenditure increased fourfold, with Viet Nam making the largest jump, from 0.83% in 1990 to 3% in 2010, followed

by Thailand, 1%–3%, while Indonesia made the smallest increase in contribution from 0.52% (1990) to 1% (2010). Again, Myanmar was the only country
with incomplete data. Cambodia's and the Philippines' proportionate spending
remained the same (see p. 55). The increase occurred across a range of different regime types, suggesting no apparent relationship between increased health
spending as a proportion of national spending and democratization. The more
autocratic Viet Nam (with a Polity score of Neg7) increased its health spending
the most, followed by Thailand (Pos4) while health spending in more democratic Indonesia (Pos8) grew the least, and in the positively correlated Cambodia (Pos2) and the Philippines (Pos8), health expenditure did not grow at
all. Likewise, Viet Nam had the largest reduction in military expenditure as a
proportion of GDP, while Indonesia's military expenditure has had the smallest
reduction.

Second, over the 20-year period studied, the region has continued its marked
decline in armed conflict. During this period, three countries secured a
cessation of hostilities and established enduring peace—Cambodia, Indonesia,
and Laos—and the Philippines may become the fourth state to achieve peace.
At the time of this writing, Myanmar is in the process of implementing a peace
process with 10 out of 18 armed groups, though intense battles and high loss of
life continues in the North and West states. In the Philippines, President Duterte
has placed Mindanao under a state of emergency rule (2017–2018) after an intense conflict with Islamist armed groups in the city of Marawi in 2017. During
the same period, Indonesia peacefully transitioned from an authoritarian to
a democratic state, and Cambodia, Myanmar, and the Philippines have held
peaceful elections (with exceptions in some localities).

Third, health trends have been positive across the region, with all countries
making improvements that range from the marginal to the dramatic. Average
life expectancy has remained lowest among the same states identified in 1990:
Myanmar (55.6 years) retains the lowest HALE in 2010, followed by Laos
(55.9 years), Cambodia (58 years), the Philippines (60.3 years), and Indonesia
(60.9 years). However, Viet Nam made one of the greatest leaps in HALE measures, from 59.5 to 65.8.

Individual DALYs for infectious diseases reveal a more complicated picture
(IHME 2013). For HIV in 1990, Thailand reported a DALY ranking worse than
the global mean, and in 2010 Myanmar was added to this list. The three countries in 1990 experiencing higher than average malaria burden among their
population improved compared to only one country (Myanmar) in 2010. TB has
consistently exacted a heavy burden in the region, with six countries having

a high DALY burden for TB—well above the global average in 1990 and continuing with five countries in 2010 (Cambodia, Indonesia, Laos, Myanmar, and the Philippines).[5] Concerning maternal complications, Cambodia, Laos, and the Philippines continued to fare worse than the global mean, while Viet Nam improved its own DALY rank in this area.

Finally, of particular interest regarding the relationship between regime type and health expenditure, there was a relatively weak trend in the region toward internal democratization. This reflects previous research noting the region's general failure to follow the presumed positive relationship between economic development and democratization (Tang 2012; for a contrasting view, see Goldsmith 2014). According to the Polity scale, four countries moved closer to democratization: with Indonesia making the most dramatic transition from Neg7 (1990) to Pos8 (2010), Myanmar made the least significant jump from Neg7 to Neg6 over the same period, and Viet Nam's score remained static over the 20 years as an autocratic regime (Neg7). In other words, the region's significant overall advances in health were made in the absence of significant democratization, and the most rapid improvements in health occurred in countries that are not democracies (Viet Nam and Singapore) or scored lower in the democratic range (Thailand at Pos4 and Malaysia at Pos6).

Southeast Asia has therefore experienced a shift of priorities in government spending, with the proportion of government spending on the military declining while the proportion spent on public health has increased (Myanmar excluded). Southeast Asia appears to confirm the importance of government investment to maintain political stability and echoes general findings concerning the positive relationship between welfare spending and its pacifying effect (Iqbal 2010; Taydas and Peksen 2012). Yet it has experienced this transformation in the absence of a concomitant democratic transition.

The five countries that increased their public health expenditure as a proportion of GDP in 2010 (see table 2.2) three democracies (Indonesia, Malaysia, and Thailand) and two nondemocracies (Laos and Viet Nam). With the exception of Singapore, the three countries that did not increase their expenditure in public health were two democracies, Cambodia and Philippines, and one nondemocracy, Myanmar. In the ASEAN case, public health investment does not seem to be dependent on democratization (Hegre 2014: 164). In fact, the outstanding performer in terms of health spending and outcomes was Viet Nam, which made no move toward democratization during the same period.

Among those listed as still experiencing low- to medium-intensity conflict in 2010, (the Philippines and Myanmar), the Philippines still scored (with

Indonesia) the highest trend toward complete democracy (Pos10). Cambodia and the Philippines are of particular interest because both are recorded as democracies in 2010, their proportionate public spending on military has declined, but their proportion of spending on health has remained lower than the proportion of GDP spent on the military, and neither country has increased health expenditure over the 20-year period (Ear 2012). Additionally, it is worth recalling that Cambodia's and the Philippines' HALE scores are among some of the lowest in the region—at the same level as Myanmar and Laos (autocracies).

Out of the 10 states, only 4 moved toward democratization over the 20-year period. Those that did so were not more likely than their nondemocratic peers to increase health expenditure as a proportion of the national budget and in preference to military expenditure. On the one hand, the democratization trend in Southeast Asia itself is not sufficiently strong to posit a connection between a particular type of regime and the generally positive health trends seen in the region. On the other, the individual results for democratizing states is mixed. This conforms with research on the weaker relationship between nascent democratization and health gains (Besley and Kudamatsu 2006; Ross 2006). Indonesia, for example, had the most significant positive change in its Polity score over the 20-year period but had one of the smallest increases in health expenditure and relatively small gains in health improvement measures. The same is true of Cambodia and the Philippines. Cambodia, 20 years on, has produced a positive but weak democracy score (Pos2) but failed to prioritize health expenditure over military expenditure as a proportion of GDP. Likewise, the Philippines has one of the strongest democracy scores (Pos8)—sustained for the 20-year period studied—but military expenditure is still marginally higher than health expenditure, and health gains have been small. In contrast, Viet Nam, which is clearly identified as an autocratic regime and consistently did not score well on the Polity scorecard (Neg7), had the largest increase in health expenditure, the largest decrease in military expenditure, and one of the largest health improvements over this period. Laos, scored as autocracy (Neg7), has a public health expenditure that is same proportion as positively scored Cambodia and Philippines. Singapore consistently scores Neg2 but has one of the highest public health expenditures as proportion of GDP, and it also has a high military expenditure, which is substantially higher than health spending. In the positive range, Thailand consistently had positive Polity scores over this period and had increased health expenditure while decreasing military expenditure. Yet life expectancy for Thailand and Viet Nam is the same

(65 years) while Malaysia—also following the expected trends of strong democracy scores, reduced military expenditure, and increased health expenditure (though less than Thailand and Viet Nam)—has a life expectancy of 64 years.

If we look at the health of the populations and take into account the political stability of these countries, there is no doubt that Ghobarah, Huth, and Russett's (2004) finding about the sustained intergenerational negative effect of armed conflict on health applies. Cambodia, Indonesia, Laos, Myanmar, and Philippines were all listed in 1990 as experiencing low to high levels of armed conflict, and their consistently lowest HALE scores in 1990 and 2010 reflect the ongoing cost of civil war to the population's health. In 2004, Ghobarah, Huth, and Russett ranked (2004: 869–884), in order, HIV, malaria, TB, and maternal complications as the principal sources of harm to postconflict populations, and, unsurprisingly, those countries in Southeast Asia with scores worse than the global mean were those that were still experiencing conflict between 1990 and 2010 (Philippines and Myanmar). The only disease among those listed where all states, except Myanmar, made improvements was malaria.

There is no doubt that the majority of ASEAN member states were in a stronger position to begin compliance work on the revised IHR than they would have been at any time prior. Since 2010, the majority of states in the region have launched universal health care, or national health insurance, schemes. However, this was a region where competing political challenges and different domestic environments were (and still are) at play. Conflict-to-postconflict transition was occurring in Myanmar and the Philippines, coupled with a relatively recent history of political transition for Cambodia, Indonesia, and Thailand. As shown, health status and health system strength sit at quite different spectrums across this region.

Since the adoption of the IHR revisions in 2005, the consistent message has been that for the instrument to work as intended there must be prompt and transparent communication among signatory states (Heymann 2006; Whelan 2008). There has been less discussion, however, of the political conditions that enable and constrain political willingness to communicate outbreak events. In the literature on this topic, public trust in the government and, in turn, the government's willingness to be transparent are identified as the key conditions necessary for any health system to meet its obligation to mount an effective first response to an outbreak emergency (Lee and Fidler 2007; O'Malley, Rainford, and Thompson 2009; Wigely and Wigely-Akkoyunlu 2011; Rockers, Kruk, and Laugesen 2012; Calain and Abu Sa'Da 2015; Desclaux, Diop, and Doyon 2017).

In 2009, O'Malley, Rainford, and Thompson argued that to progress IHR compliance, public trust in the government and transparent governance processes were vital in order to implement IHR core capacities such as surveillance, response, and risk communication. They defined transparency as reflecting two aspects specific to the IHR: the quality of information and communication from the government to the public, and public trust in government communication and decisions (O'Malley, Rainford, and Thompson 2009). In the case of the IHR, surveillance and response as well as risk communication are the areas identified as the core capacity preconditions for the IHR to achieve what was intended in 2005—to communicate outbreak events promptly and effectively.

The conditions necessary for these two aspects of transparency depend upon having a health system that is trusted, which depends upon public trust in the government. Rockers, Kruk, and Laugesen (2012) argue that health system performance and public trust in governance are strongly interrelated in low- and middle-income countries. Wigley and Akkoyunlu-Wigley (2011) argue that media freedoms are closely connected to regime type, and democracies are more likely to uphold media freedoms, which, in turn, enhance citizens' trust in health messages. Desclaux, Diop, and Doyon (2017: 212) point to a critical relationship among trust, politics, and securitization. The Ebola outbreak in West Africa revealed how the absence of public trust in a government created the need for "authoritarian interventions by government security decisions makers" to ensure compliance, which further heightened public fear (and resistance).

The research above suggests that a political environment receptive to IHR reform is as important as meeting the technical and financial goals (Calain and Sa'Da 2015). The IHR reforms certainly require technical proficiency, but they also take place in a political environment. What is less clear is the type of political environment necessary for IHR reform matters. Aside from direct appeals to a state, which may or may not work, can regional coordination and cooperation provide a middle path?

The remainder of this book seeks to understand why and how one region, despite great variation in health, socioeconomic, and political contexts, sought to achieve IHR reform as a collective regional exercise in its first phase of introduction.

Conclusion

When it comes to the politics of health, political systems matter. The allocation of public resources to health care can lead to improvements in health and is a means to sustain peace and stability. To date, the key point of departure for explaining why some governments prioritize health and others do not has been the role of democracy. Democracy pushes regimes to prioritize welfare spending and therefore democracy may produce improved health outcomes such as greater compliance with the IHR. However, the Southeast Asian experience suggests that the relationship between political systems and health systems is more complex. Understanding this relationship is vital to discern whether regime type compromises compliance with the IHR. This is a theme I return to in chapter 6 in analyzing how individual ASEAN states have realized their surveillance and response obligations under the IHR.

The following chapter turns to how and why Southeast Asian states came to appreciate the management of infectious disease as a collective obligation. From 2000 onward, addressing disease outbreaks and linking their containment to effective national health capacity has had an increasingly receptive audience in Southeast Asia. By the time of the SARS and H5N1 outbreaks in the region, what had become contentious was whether this promotion of health security would be at the cost of local needs with existing health burdens and health inequalities.

CHAPTER THREE

Sovereignty, Regional Cooperation, and Health Security

In 2007, the WHO annual report on the state of global health observed that a pandemic influenza event was inevitable at some point and most likely to occur in Asia (WHO 2007b). Following the outbreak of SARS in the first half of 2003, a H5N1 avian influenza outbreak was identified in poultry in East Asia in November 2003. Then cases of human infection with H5N1 appeared in 2004, with nearly all cases of human infection resulting from direct contact with poultry. What was so concerning about the reemergence of H5N1 (first detected in Hong Kong in 1997) was that "H5N1 infection in humans results in about 60% mortality among confirmed cases, yet it is only sporadically transmitted to humans and even less often between humans. [Yet w]hen thinking about a potential H5N1 pandemic, large numbers of fatalities could be assumed because the virus had proved itself to be highly lethal" (WHA 2011: 11). These events, coupled with an increasing incidence of region-wide dengue, enterovirus (hand, foot, and mouth disease), and Japanese encephalitis outbreaks, have no doubt led to Southeast Asia being identified as a potential "hot zone" for emerging infectious diseases (Jones et al. 2008; Coker et al. 2011).

In this chapter, I examine how infectious disease outbreak events in the region attracted "securitized" responses from Southeast Asian states and how this normative framing of infectious diseases influenced states' approaches to the revised IHR. The chapter shows that recognition of a collective sense of health insecurity in the region played a crucial role in establishing a common interest that helped support the generation of trust sufficient to ensure regional cooperation on disease surveillance and core capacities. The adoption of the overarching international framework to which these member states are bound—the revised International Health Regulations (2005)—was the result of a regional process of deepening disease detection and reporting platforms that built upon already existing layers of thought, practice, and cooperation among the ASEAN membership.

I chronicle the securitization of infectious disease among the ASEAN membership and show how the obligation to recognize infectious disease outbreak as a shared threat was impressed upon states and societies, irrespective of their political type or health system capacity (Calain 2007). The chapter proceeds in three parts. First, it recounts how regional threats—SARS and H5N1 in particular—shaped regional interpretations of the IHR negotiations and the subsequent core capacity requirements. Occurring at the same time as the IHR negotiations, the H5N1 outbreak in Indonesia, Thailand, and Viet Nam revealed crucial internal weaknesses in national health systems and created internal demands for reform compatible with the emerging global agenda. The second part of the chapter details how Southeast Asian states came to understand these events in increasingly securitized terms and the different types of political arrangements that developed in response. The final part of the chapter argues that it was the combination of these events and ASEAN's prior commitment to a securitized understanding of health that created its receptiveness to APSED. The chapter briefly introduces APSED and the articulation of its purpose in the first phase as promoting national and regional capacity-building objectives in two critical areas: combatting infectious diseases as a regional security threat and enhancing national-level expertise across the IHR core capacities.

This chapter argues that the securitization of disease outbreaks in the region sharpened the focus of the early stages of the APSED project, particularly its contribution to disease outbreak surveillance and response (Horby, Pfeiffer, and Oshitani 2013: 858), which is further discussed in chapter 4. Infectious disease surveillance outbreak and response became a primary focus for regional- and state-level engagement with the IHR (Ijaz et al. 2012; WHO 2014). As this chapter and the chapters that follow reveal, surveillance and response was a primary objective in the first phase of APSED. States risked characterization as irresponsible, even a source of the insecurity to the region, if they did not participate in the revised IHR process. This language was particularly powerful, given the capacity-building project being undertaken within ASEAN at the time.

Cumulative Effect of SARS and H5N1: The Revised IHR and ASEAN States

The shock of the SARS outbreak proved to be a crucial global event that contributed to the final agreement on the IHR in 2005. The relatively low transmissibility of the virus and the infectious period of the disease, along with the relatively simple public health measures required to contain it (isolation and quarantining their contacts), meant that the disease did not spread as rapidly as it might have (Anderson et al. 2003: 76). The SARS virus was eventually declared contained by the WHO after approximately 8,400 infections and 774 deaths on 5 July 2003. A delay in verifying the outbreak in China initially inhibited efforts to contain the spread of the disease. However, the surprising strength of the system proved to be the WHO's coordinated response with its regional offices and associated collaborating laboratories—which led to the isolation of a new virus within three months and the deployment of multinational fieldwork teams in greatly affected Hong Kong, Viet Nam, and (eventually) China.

Moreover, "countries did not refuse to report or collaborate on the grounds that SARS (and most other infectious diseases) was not covered by the International Health Regulations (1969)" (Heymann 2006: 352). There was little open criticism by states of the role that the WHO played during the SARS outbreak (Fidler 2004a: 188–189). As such, immediately after SARS, the WHO maintained that the key lesson was that delays in verification inhibit efforts to stem the spread of infectious disease. The WHO's authority to monitor disease outbreaks and issue travel advisories could not effectively stem outbreaks unless it had some authority to demand state cooperation (Heymann and Rodier 2004). This was the "tipping point" for the IHR revisions (Davies, Kamradt-Scott, and Rushton 2015).

In the aftermath of SARS and the IHR (2005) revisions, the WHO argued in the 2007 *World Health Report* that "in an electronically transparent world where outbreaks are particularly newsworthy events, their concealment is no longer a viable option for governments" (WHO 2007b: 13). At the time, WHO assistant director-general David Heymann and WHO director of Communicable Disease Unit Guénaël Rodier maintained that "inadequate surveillance and response capacity in a single country can endanger national populations and the public health security of the entire world. As long as national capacities are weak, international mechanisms for outbreak alert and response will be needed" (2004: 173). The revised IHR (2005) thus required that all states develop, in particular, an internal surveillance and outbreak response capacity (WHO 2007a: 15–16).

To further complicate matters, at the time that the SARS outbreak was occupying global attention, H5N1 was making its reentrance (H5N1 was first detected in Hong Kong in 1997). By the beginning of 2004, H5N1 poultry infections had led to the first wave of serious H5N1 human infections, with China, Viet Nam, and Thailand all confirming cases of human infection (Morris and Jackson 2005: 15–19). By June 2004, Indonesia, Cambodia, and Laos confirmed their first cases of poultry infections, while Thailand started to experience its second wave of H5N1 infections in poultry and humans. H5N1 was first identified in poultry in South Korea in December 2003. In the same month, Thailand raised the alarm when the H5N1 virus strain was discovered in sick tigers and leopards in the Bangkok Zoo, which was traced to infected poultry in their diet.

When Viet Nam reported its first H5N1 human case, there were fears that the disease had already adapted to human transmission when a cluster of cases from one family was identified there in February 2004 (Writing Committee of the WHO Consultation on Human Influenza A 2005). In the same month Thailand reported its first two human infections (direct from poultry). By the end of 2004, Viet Nam and Thailand confirmed six and five human infection cases, respectively. By 2005, Cambodia, China, and Indonesia had confirmed cases of H5N1 human infections, and, at the end of the same year, Indonesia had the highest human caseload of infections, with 20 cases (WHO 2011). To get a sense of how serious the potential threat was, the fatality rate for humans infected with H5N1 was 73% in 2004, 63% in 2005, and 43% in 2006. Moreover, 90% of cases were in people under the age of 40 (Writing Committee of the Second WHO Consultation on Clinical Aspects of Human Infection with Avian Influenza [H5N1] Virus 2008).

By the end of 2006, Indonesia still had the highest human caseload of infections, with 55 cases and 45 deaths (WHO 2011); and, by 2008, the virus had spread to wild birds and domestic poultry across the Middle East, North Africa, West Africa, Eastern and Western Europe, and South Asia. Within Asia, Myanmar (where the first known human case was reported in December 2007), Japan, and the Republic of Korea were now reporting seasonal outbreaks in poultry. In 2008, the WHO estimated the H5N1 human infection case fatality rate was 60% but was still reporting no sustained, successful local transmission of the virus between humans (Writing Committee of the Second WHO Consultation on Clinical Aspects of Human Infection with Avian Influenza [H5N1] Virus 2008).

At the same time, to varying degrees, scientists started to voice concern that China, Thailand, and Viet Nam were too slow in reporting H5N1 outbreaks (Ear 2010; Forster 2010; Safman 2010; Vu 2010). The worry was that the state-level response to H5N1—despite the adoption of the revised IHR occurring at the same time—was being affected by a reluctance to invite international assistance, delay in reporting detections, and inconsistent risk communication practices at the local level. However, not all agreed with this characterization of affected states' responses. Some pointed out that Asian states were complying with the intended spirit of the revised IHR even though the instrument and its core capacities had not yet come into force (Lee and Fidler 2007: 220). David Heymann went so far as to argue that "Asian governments continued to adhere to the norms and standards that had been established during the SARS outbreak by open reporting of, and collaborative response to, important events in public health [such as H5N1]" (2006: 352).

At the outset of the H5N1 outbreak, there was no formal requirement for states to report and verify the disease since the revised IHR had not yet been adopted. The WHO was quick to suggest that the lack of a formal reporting requirement had inhibited the response but should not prevent cooperation in practice. The WHO, with the UN Food and Agriculture Organization (FAO) and World Organization for Animal Health, issued a joint statement in January 2004 calling for cooperation and for funding to assist governments in containment (FAO/WHO 2004). As the rate of infections rose over 2004 and 2006, the outbreak was consistently identified as a threat that required extraordinary dedication of both cooperation and resources (FAO/WHO 2004; ASEAN 2006: 1).

The position adopted by ASEAN was similar to the WHO's: member states had a duty to report, but the ASEAN secretariat and its member states made it clear international assistance should follow international attention to Asia's H5N1 response. At this juncture, the ASEAN position on H5N1 being reported as if the revised IHR applied was significant for two reasons. First, many of its member states were among those most affected by the H5N1 outbreak and would have to comply with reporting expectations; and, second, the ASEAN secretariat was quite proactive in promoting the role of the WHO in assisting its member states and in promoting the need for shared outbreak communication between states and the WHO (Pitsuwan 2011). The first high-level ministry meetings organized to discuss the collective response to H5N1 was the APT Health Ministers Meeting on Avian Influenza in Bangkok, Thailand, in November 2004. At this meeting, the "Joint Ministerial Statement on Prevention and Control of Avian Influenza, Bangkok, Thailand"—26 November 2004—was adopted:

> We commit ourselves, in view of the changing circumstances:
>   *to facilitate prompt and open exchange of information on avian influenza between nations and with concerned international agencies with the view to ensure transparency, facilitate consultation and fair application of health-related measures of international concern especially during outbreaks;*

to take the necessary steps to develop and implement effective national influenza pandemic preparedness plans;

to further strengthen and harmonize activities related to all important aspects of Avian Influenza, including surveillance, investigation of cases, characterization of the epidemiology of the disease, defining appropriate public health responses;

to collaborate in the effort for the development of vaccines, diagnostic tests for human disease and promoting other appropriate research activities. As part of these efforts, to facilitate the provision of virus isolates to the relevant laboratory networks to allow optimal vaccine strain selection;

to collaborate with relevant agencies and sectors in promoting food safety and safe animal husbandry practices with the aim of minimizing human health risks;

to further intensify efforts to make resources available to address this *public health threat.*

We request WHO, in collaboration with relevant international organizations,

to support the implementation of our commitments notably the collaborative researches, and the strengthening of the preparedness for the influenza pandemic;

to establish bi-regional effective mechanism in supporting the sustainable implementation of the collaborative efforts among countries, including the control of other emerging infectious diseases;

to facilitate global and regional collaboration to make available the resources required to combat this public health threat, especially for developing countries without sufficient resources. (APT Joint Statement 2004; emphasis added)

Individual states were, however, increasingly affected by the outbreak, struggling in both technical capacity (i.e., Viet Nam) and government willingness to report cases (i.e., Thailand) (Thomas 2006). Significantly and in direct response, regional collaboration was further deepened by the ASEAN secretariat and its member states, establishing in October 2004 an ASEAN Highly Pathogenic Avian Influenza (HPAI) Taskforce to assist member states in containment measures to control the disease in the domestic, industry, and wildlife animal sectors (UNSIC 2011: 7). APT also issued support for the creation of the ASEAN HPAI Taskforce and agreed to provide expertise and assistance (UNSIC 2011: 6). Within a year, by September 2005, the HPAI Taskforce received member state endorsement of the Regional Framework for Control and Eradication of Highly Pathogenic Avian Influenza. This came three months after the revised IHR had been adopted and well before they came into force in 2007.

The HPAI framework covered "eight (8) strategic areas on the prevention, control and eradication of HPAI over a period of three years (2006 to 2008), under the coordination of assigned Member Countries" (ASEAN 2006: 2) and included

(i) Disease surveillance—coordinated by Thailand;

(ii) Effective containment measures—coordinated by Malaysia;

(iii) Stamping out and vaccination policy—coordinated by Indonesia;

(iv) Diagnostic capabilities—coordinated by Thailand;

(v) Establishment of disease free zones—coordinated by Malaysia;

(vi) Information sharing—coordinated by Singapore;

(vii) Emergency Preparedness Plans—coordinated by Malaysia; and

(viii) Public Awareness—coordinated by the Philippines. (ASEAN 2006: 2)

China agreed to host, on behalf of the APT group, an International Pledging Conference on Avian and Human Influenza in Beijing on 17–18 January 2006. Multiple bilateral and multilateral funding partnerships developed from the Beijing pledging conference, with major donors including the European Union, World Bank, Asian Development Bank, the US Centers for Disease Control and Prevention, China CDC, Japan-ASEAN Integration Fund, AusAID, and the Public Health Agency of Canada (ASEAN 2006: 2).

In 2006, despite these efforts, human H5N1 cases dramatically increased, especially in Viet Nam and Indonesia. The WHA-adopted Resolution WHA59.2 (2006) urged all member states to implement on a voluntary basis the IHR (2005) in response to the threat posed by avian influenza (WHA 2006). As David Fidler and Lawrence Gostin (2008: 246) argue, Resolution WHA59.2 not only demonstrated the degree to which states appreciated the risk of (and their vulnerability to) the avian influenza outbreak, it also revealed political commitment to revisions (and the core capacities) that did not to come into force until June 2007. Significantly, the ASEAN secretariat again iterated a collective political commitment in a statement issued in April 2006:

From the experience with SARS in 2003, ASEAN learned that an effective means of prevention is to ensure our peoples are better informed on the causes of the disease, its main modes of transmission and preventive steps to take. Providing researchers and public information bodies with prompt, transparent and reliable information on avian influenza occurrences (either in poultry or human) is critical in lessening public fear of the virus. ASEAN overcame SARS by acting with transparency. Timely information was provided on preventive measures. Strict quarantine and monitoring measures were instituted. New equipment and technology for thermal screening at exit and entry points were shared freely. Hotlines were activated to ensure quick information-sharing. Therefore, sharing information, knowledge, success stories and lessons learned from each specific case experienced thus far will help institute better preparedness, surveillance and testing procedures in animal and human health systems. (ASEAN 2006: 3)

Between 2007 and 2008, the H5N1 human infections (and poultry cases) were gradually brought under control. Cases continued to be reported in Egypt, Indonesia, Cambodia, Viet Nam, and China (in order of prevalence up to the end of 2010) (WHO 2011). During this period, the virus did not mutate to become the pandemic influenza many feared (ASEAN 2012a: 708). Many have since interpreted the Southeast Asian regional response to H5N1 as indicating some success in individual state and international efforts to collaboratively combat emerging infectious diseases (Wilsmore et al. 2010). However, attention primarily focused on the controversy over virus sharing that arose during the H5N1 outbreak and the perception that therefore affected states like Indonesia, Viet Nam, and Thailand were also opposing the revised IHR, even the language of global health security (Calain 2007; Aldis 2008).

There were disincentives to reporting H5N1. First, governments were not legally required to report to the WHO or anyone else for the first three and a half years of the H5N1 outbreak (Lee and Fidler 2007: 220). Even under WHA59.2, the extent of states' obligation was a voluntary commitment to report H5N1 outbreaks. Second, the financial costs associated with confirming an H5N1 outbreak, especially the destruction of poultry stocks and associated farming livelihoods, were a major deterrent to report (Thomas 2006; Forster 2010; Safman 2010). The three leading poultry producers, Indonesia, Thailand, and Viet Nam, faced significant losses to their GDP. In 2010, the cost of the H5N1 outbreak within six years had been 200 million poultry culled and a collective US$10 billion in economic losses (McKenna 2010). Third, as discussed in chapter 2, the strength and capacity of health and political systems varied across the region—and those states most affected by H5N1. They faced multiple stressors on their capacity, which affected their willingness at times to report early and correctly (S. Davies 2012). At the front of this response were the public health responders and the bureaucrats responsible for policy advice and implementation. Pressures of public anxiety, the need to reassure societies about the measures that governments were taking, media interest, and political machinations attached to outbreak response resulted in difficult decision-making environments for public health workers, who had to balance their capacity to diagnose accurately with their obligation to report and face the political and economic implications of their reports.

However, the rapid coordination of a regional response to the H5N1 outbreak—given the newness of the revised IHR—was organized around a logic of responding to emerging disease outbreaks, and it had been developing for some time. The fear of an uncontrolled outbreak compelled cooperation and normalized the expectation of regional reporting, sharing information, and acting as a coordinated group. In the next section, I briefly examine how and why ASEAN came to approach emerging infectious diseases as a matter of *regional security*. Then I turn to how this understanding informed states' commitment to the revised IHR, their reporting performance, and the development of APSED.

ASEAN's Normative Role

Within the field of international relations, ASEAN is probably best known as a regional organization for its lack of formal institutions that bind states to compromise the principle of sovereign noninterference (Johnston 2012; Goldsmith 2014). Since its creation in 1967, the Association of Southeast Asian Nations (founding members Indonesia, Malaysia, Philippines, Singapore, and Thailand; then Brunei [Darussalam] in 1984; Viet Nam in 1995; Lao PDR [Laos] and Myanmar in 1997; and Cambodia in 1999), has primarily dedicated itself to the preservation of peace and security in the region through establishing a very strict interpretation of sovereignty. The 1976 Treaty of Amity and Cooperation (TAC) remains the key instrument fundamental to ASEAN practice (Ba 2009):

1. Mutual respect for the independence, sovereignty, equality, territorial integrity, and national identity of all nations
2. The right of every state to lead its national existence free from external interference, subversion or coercion
3. Noninterference in the internal affairs of one another
4. Settlement of differences or disputes by peaceful manner
5. Renunciation of the threat or use of force
6. Effective cooperation among themselves

To this day, TAC is the instrument all states must sign if they wish to engage in formal membership or partnership with ASEAN. In 1997, China, Japan, and South Korea signed TAC to form APT. Likewise, Australia, New Zealand, the United States, and Russia have signed TAC to participate in ASEAN's annual East Asia Summit. In the 2008 ASEAN Charter, TAC is referred to as embodying the "traditional state-centered norms of ASEAN" (Morada 2009: 196).

The creation of the charter and its entry into force in 2009 marked a shift from ASEAN's history of soft institutionalization with minimal imposition on sovereignty. Events and policies from the charter itself indicate this shift. For example, in the same year the charter was adopted, ASEAN secretariat persuaded the Myanmar government to accept international humanitarian assistance after the Cyclone Nargis disaster. ASEAN secretary-general Surin Pitsuwan, along with one of the ASEAN founding members, Indonesia, took an active diplomatic role in persuading Myanmar that refusal of assistance based on the principle of "sovereign non-interference" was harming the civilian population and the credibility of ASEAN (Haacke 2009: 173). This event presents, some have argued, a changed understanding of TAC and its invulnerability to events that test the responsibility of states to protect their civilian population against the principle of sovereign noninterference (Caballero-Antony 2008).

The adoption of the ASEAN Charter also presages the formalization of an ASEAN regional identity (Ba 2009: 7). While the normative superiority of the sovereign state has not been threatened by the 2008 charter, it is true that increasingly regional unity (regionalism) has come to be seen as an "answer to important security challenges" (Ba 2009: 7). From transboundary haze to maritime piracy, ASEAN member states have a tradition of turning to the institution when addressing nontraditional security challenges that threaten, heedless of borders and political regimes (Callabero-Anthony and Emmers 2006). Securitization in the ASEAN context has multiple meanings and approaches, but the consistency in the ASEAN context is that it has rarely challenged the state-centered concept of security (Foot 2014: 199–200). Securitization of infectious disease, as with piracy, migration, and pollution, meet the "comprehensive security" approach of ASEAN states, which is regime legitimization and survival (Acharya 2006: 249). Regional responses are often presented as a "dialogue" and "consensus" in public statements; even newly created regional institutions such as the ASEAN Intergovernmental Commission on Human Rights have been described as a forum where rhetoric is strong but institutional reinforcement is weak (M. Davies 2013). No doubt, despite the creation of the ASEAN

Charter and its associated commissions and committees, there remains a reluctance to vest too much power in regional institutions at the cost of state
autonomy (Foot 2014: 206).

However, ASEAN's underlying principle of sovereign noninterference does
not preclude the opportunity for regional initiatives that encourage state-level
cooperation that challenges the preservation of the noninterference norm
(Haacke and Williams 2008; Acharya 2009; Caballero-Anthony 2014). Alice
Ba (2009) argues that ASEAN's continued presence and institutional expansion
(in membership, charter, and institutions) is the product of a four-decade
history of careful negotiation of nationalism with regionalism through a process of argumentation, consensus, and dialogue (Ba 2009: 10). The absence of
formal institutionalism to enforce agreements means that looking at material
forces and strategic bargaining will not explain the normative dynamics of
ASEAN (Acharya 2009: 152). We must trace the soft and nonlegalistic engagement, the social arrangements, and the history of a "common interpretation of
problems" to understand ASEAN's persuasive power (Ba 2009: 12). Ba argues,
in fact, that, because of the dominance of sovereign noninterference in ASE-
AN's formal relations, we tend to overlook the transformative work achieved
through the informal practices within the institution: "Academic and policy
discourses sometimes can overly downplay these kinds of contributions—
which ultimately are associated with ASEAN's role in shaping the social environment of cooperation, but are arguably just as important as any specific
'functional cooperation' and, as suggested, may even be considered a precondition of such cooperation" (Ba 2010: 127–128).

If we accept Ba's argument that ASEAN's informal cooperative structure
creates a social environment of cooperation, the purpose of articulating infectious disease outbreaks as a security concern for all ASEAN member states—
regardless of health system capacity—becomes clear. Promoting infectious
disease to the status of a "common regional problem" required dialogue and
unity in prioritizing coordinated disease outbreak surveillance and response
procedures. It is true, as others have pointed out, that we cannot observe the
creation of formal procedures around notification of particular diseases or preparedness at the ASEAN level (Haacke and Williams 2008; Stevenson and
Cooper 2009; Lamy and Phua 2012; Kamradt-Scott, Lee, and Xu 2013).

Individual states still exercise primary control over health funding and its
distribution (which varies, as chap. 2 showed). Securitization of infectious
disease can and has produced negative consequences for those infected with
diseases such as HIV within the region (Ramiah 2006), and the way bureaucrats

must meet the 24/7 reporting conditions laid out in the revised IHR often remains opaque when under the control of highly centralized executive governments like Cambodia, Myanmar, and Viet Nam. Despite these facts, as I show in chapters 5 and 6, there is *near* uniformity in how states have changed their surveillance and response functions over time, especially since the introduction of the revised IHR, that illustrates individual states are making efforts to meet the regional expectation of improved detection and response. Given the outbreaks occurring in the region, the political and economic disincentives, and the capacity shortfalls, progress could not have been assumed or predicted in 2005. Therefore, what regional discussions took place in the first phase of the revised IHR's adoption and implementation? The ASEAN secretariat promoted from the outset social networks among the membership to discuss and support implementation of the revised IHR at the state level (Caballero-Anthony et al. 2015).

Health as a Nontraditional Security Threat to ASEAN States

ASEAN's regional institution and the policy implementation demanded from its membership have undergone dramatic shifts since its creation in 1967 and the adoption of TAC in 1976. The 2008 ASEAN Charter was an ambitious project in many respects for 10 states so committed to the principle of noninterference. The charter outlines a "firm foundation in achieving the ASEAN Community by providing legal status and institutional framework for ASEAN. It also codifies ASEAN norms, rules and values; sets clear targets for ASEAN; and presents accountability and compliance" (ASEAN 2008). The 2008 charter committed to the professionalization of the ASEAN secretariat and permitted the adoption of regional legal instruments on shared economic zones, migration, financial transactions, and human rights. New regional bodies like the ASEAN Intergovernmental Commission on Human Rights and the ASEAN Coordinating Centre for Humanitarian Assistance on disaster management has followed. However—unlike the African Union and European Union—the 2008 charter did not inspire the creation of a supranational assembly, council, court, or parliament where shared laws and actions may be passed and possibly enforced against the wishes of another member state (Acharya 2004: 146; also Haacke and Morada 2010).

The incremental changes within the charter came in the wake of some ASEAN members' individual paths toward democratization, particularly among founding members Indonesia, Philippines, and Thailand. The pursuit of economic growth and regional stability to optimize that growth has also inspired regional coordination on policies that are more human centered than state centered (Tan 2011; Goldsmith 2013).

Issues, policies, and events scheduled under the ASEAN community's three pillars—political-security, economy, and sociocultural—have become an important barometer of the region's collective thinking on any particular issue. While the ASEAN community projects the pillars as equal, it is informally understood that the sociocultural, where the health issues, policy, and ministerial meetings reside, receives the least attention and political investment of the three pillars (Pitsuwan 2011; Davies, Nackers, and Teitt 2014; Amaya, Rollet, and Kingah 2015). Even at the strongest point of securitization language in response to health threats, namely outbreaks of infectious disease in the region, ASEAN's consideration of health issues has remained under the Socio-Cultural Community (specifically under the purview of the ASEAN Health Ministers Meeting [AHMM], which meets biannually under the Socio-Cultural Community Council; ASEAN 2012a). During the height of the H5N1 outbreak, there was never any move to permanently shift even the topic of infectious disease response (for example) from AHMM to the ASEAN Political-Security Community (Haacke and Williams 2008). Indeed, Mely Caballero-Anthony (2008) has argued that, despite the region engaging with health as a nontraditional security threat from the 1990s in informal political-security discussions, efforts to develop a formal high-level process did not really emerge until after the SARS and H5N1 outbreak (Caballero-Anthony and Amul 2014: 39).

SARS, followed by H5N1, attracted a lot of attention to the region's capacity to respond to emerging infectious disease threats, but this was not the region's first confrontation with a novel infectious disease outbreak or outbreaks on a regional scale. In 1998 the region experienced the threat of Nipah virus, which originated from the farmed pig population in Malaysia and went on to infect humans, spreading to Singapore in 1999. Endemic diseases such as enterovirus (hand, foot, and mouth disease), dengue, and its deadlier relative, dengue hemorrhagic fever (DHF), have also become regular seasonal fixtures in most ASEAN countries due to a combination of climate change (rising temperatures), migration, and rapid urbanization. Japanese encephalitis and malaria were (and still are) becoming harder to combat in the region, with increased urbanization, confined living quarters between animals and humans, and extreme weather patterns (WPRO 2005; Coker et al. 2011). These experiences had already created rising concern for advisors (to ASEAN) and commentators about the ability of some ASEAN states to respond to effectively to infectious disease outbreaks, given the pronounced diversity in health system capacity, public health expenditure, and existing disease burdens (ASEAN 2012b; Caballero-Anthony et al. 2015; Kumaresan and Huikuri 2015). This concern was one that had already been identified and acted upon in the creation of subregional voluntary cooperation programs in disease outbreak reporting and response, such as the Mekong Basin Disease Surveillance (MBDS) Network among Myanmar, China, Thailand, Cambodia, Viet Nam, and Laos (Kimball et al. 2008; Phommasack et al. 2013).

In response to SARS, and then H5N1, ASEAN member states increasingly engaged in high-level (executive leadership–level) discussions that led to statements recognizing emerging infectious diseases as securitized threats (ASEAN 2003a, 2003b; APT 2004; ASEAN 2006, 2007, 2011, 2012a, 2012b, 2016). Haacke and Williams (2008) went so far as to argue that securitization in the context of ASEAN's approach to novel infectious diseases had been "successful." This judgment was made on the basis of, first, ASEAN's leadership agreeing to the identification of infectious diseases as a security threat to individual states and the wider region. This became a repeated reference in ASEAN statements (see references above). Second, the prevention and response program to SARS, then H5N1, was linked to building longer-term regional capacity to detect and respond to future outbreaks. Significantly, ASEAN's outreach was not only to the WHO for advice and assistance but also to traditional security and economic partners such as the APT and Asia-Pacific Economic Cooperation (ASEAN 2003b).

In addition to the existing AHMM and ASEAN Senior Officials Meeting on Health Development came Malaysia's hosting of the 2003 SARS Conference; the ASEAN Expert Group on Communicable Diseases; followed by the APT Emerging Infectious Diseases Programme endorsed by the ASEAN Expert Group on Communicable Diseases in 2004; the ASEAN HPAI Task Force; the Asian Development Bank grant for combating avian and human pandemic influenza in Asia and the Pacific Region; and, of course, APSED (UNSIC 2011; ASEAN 2012b).

That most of these initiatives were introduced after SARS was no accident. The SARS outbreak had significant economic, social, and political effects across Southeast Asia. There was no sector left unaffected by SARS, and for the first time "competition within the ASEAN states shifted to concern about how to collectively survive" within this new threat environment (Anonymous 2012d, 2012f).

In spite of a rapid succession of regional moves, concern remained that the response was still limited and conventional (Fidler 2013: 212). The securitization of novel infectious diseases in Asia was limited to raising awareness that these outbreaks required action on the part of the affected state to minimize its impact across the wider region (Chalk 2006; Ramiah 2006; Haacke and Williams 2008). A recurrent concern was that the securitization of infectious disease within ASEAN had (just) reinforced the idea that sovereign borders and the economy were in need of protection from disease outbreaks rather than the population (Calain 2007; Aldis 2008; Amaya, Rollet, and Kingah 2015).

Securitization certainly has multiple effects, and not all of them positive. On the one hand, securitizing infectious diseases had just strengthened conventional state practice—emphasis on containment requires a state to be seen to be doing "something" whether that something is relevant or justified (Lee and Fidler 2007). The concern with this response is an increased risk of reinforcing noninterference as the primary foundation for international engagement. In the case of surveillance and response, protecting the sovereign could be seen as justifying emergency rule—controlling the flow of people and information through quarantine and limits on communication (Davies and Youde 2012). Securitization could lead to less openness and cooperation among states (O'Malley, Rainford, and Thompson 2009; Stevenson and Cooper 2009). Thus, intense securitization of novel infectious disease outbreaks within the region may be the means by which the region's states are actually preserving noninterference. Stefan Elbe (2010) argues, regarding the case of the Indonesian government's refusal in 2007 to share H5N1 virus samples with the WHO Global Influenza Surveillance Network Collaborating Centers, that securitization language was used as a context for establishing the unprecedented step of prioritizing sovereignty over viruses. The Indonesian government argued in 2007 that the current virus-sharing system left the government sharing the virus with no benefits in terms of purchasing power when a foreign company and country produces the costly vaccine (Supari 2008). The sovereign move to "own" a virus was a novel political development that had never been asserted before in the scientific field of virus sharing post–World War II (Elbe 2010). The sovereign claim over samples marked out the (re)affirmation of the sovereign— and pitched it directly against the efforts by the WHO to promote political cooperation above sovereign self-interest.

For all the talk of securitization being beneficial to the global effort to deal with infectious disease, this was seen as the proof of its potentially pernicious use (Hameiri 2014). There was little objection by ASEAN to Indonesia's move. Some states tacitly endorsed Indonesia's actions (Thailand and Viet Nam, for example), while others if they disagreed (e.g., Singapore), contributed little to the public argument (Aldis 2008). This has been regarded as evidence that any regional progress on deepening the international obligation to report and share outbreaks will remain a far distant second to sovereign interest (Stevenson and Cooper 2009).

On the other hand, it should not be assumed that securitization was the inevitable path in this case. As Buzan, Weaver, and de Wilde note in their study, what is interesting about securitization is *when* it occurs—"the attribution of security problems to specific sources rather than actual origins of what appear as security problems." A regional practice of securitization is, structurally, quite different from the unit—state-level—analysis. Buzan, Weaver, and de Wilde note that, when observing the process of securitization at the regional level, the study of the process needs to be trained on the "nodes that are simultaneously that which is (claimed to be) threatened and that which is (depicted as) the source of threat" (1998: 44).

Aligning the sovereign obligation to report an infectious disease outbreak in the name of upholding a subfield of security, that is, health security, allowed the adoption of new reporting measures without any great realignment of international norms surrounding sovereignty and disease response (Haacke and Williams 2008; Price-Smith 2009). In this instance, the degree to which subregional and regional reporting arrangements hold member states accountable to the IHR revisions may remain limited (Fidler 2013). In a situation when reporting delays are expected, highlighting regional obligations in spite of capacity constraints is a strategic move by some states in anticipation of other members trying to avoid their obligation (S. Davies 2012). Moreover, if sovereign noninterference is the only force that mobilizes state response, presenting health as a security threat to the sovereign may be the only way to assert the health rights of individuals.

The question then is, has the right tool been selected for the job? Is the attribution of infectious disease outbreaks to a security threat likely to generate sustained economic investment and political interest (Calain 2007; Aldis 2008; Caballero-Anthony 2008; Fidler 2013)? Crossing the Rubicon in this instance is the shift from comfortable use of rhetoric to investment and performance in health systems to improve detection, response, and containment (Coker et al. 2011). Specific to Southeast Asia, the focus has been on whether investment in the resources necessary to detect and report novel infectious diseases will come at the possible cost of detecting and treating diseases that the region already experience on annual basis (endemic outbreaks) (Calain 2007; Aldis 2008). Examples include Cambodia, with a reporting system in place for H5N1 human infections (five outbreaks between 2006 and 2010) but no equivalent reporting system for human Japanese encephalitis infections (estimated to have an annual caseload in the hundreds given the caseload in surrounding countries) (Ear 2010; Coker et al. 2011: 605). Donor-driven concerns with pandemic influenza in the region have been attributed to the political backlash from Thailand at the World Health Assembly immediately after the adoption of the IHR (Aldis 2008; Elbe 2010). Thailand objected to the use of "global health security," arguing that this wording is far from reconciled in the minds of many states both in terms of its resource demand and policy implications. Indonesia made similar objections to the phrase (see below) when facing critique for failing to provide samples of its H5N1 virus to the WHO influenza network. This political backlash would not be surprising for Haacke and Williams (2008), Elbe (2010), or Fidler (2013): they predicted that the "securitization-lite" framework applied to communicable disease in the region was going to produce tensions when the rhetoric then demanded specific response and action from states.

In the immediate instance, these concerns are true. However, a longer time frame sees the region persistently moving in a health securitization direction and consistently using the phrase "health security" for a wider range of health matters (Caballero-Anthony et al. 2015). The region has been a persistent presence at US-funded Global Health Security Agenda (GHSA; in place since 2014) events, and, prior to GHSA, Thailand was a participant and Indonesia was a cochair to the Norwegian Oslo Initiative on Global Health Security in 2007, which led to the first UN General Assembly resolution on global health and foreign policy in 2009 (UNGA 2009). This resolution and successive resolutions have referred to health security in the context of the Millennium Development Goals (in 2009), health care worker resourcing (UNGA 2010), health system strengthening (UNGA 2011), natural disasters (UNGA 2012), and universal health care coverage (UNGA 2013). It is worth noting that four ASEAN members (Indonesia, Philippines, Thailand, and Viet Nam) are members of the WHO–World Bank Universal Health Care Coverage Study Series formed after the 2013 resolution (Cotlear et al. 2015). Programs within the ASEAN EID and APT EID continue to meet annually to promote the programs and use the wording "health security" and "health threats" (ASEAN 2016). The ASEAN political-security committee has, when making reference to infectious diseases, continued to use the phrase "health security," and the wording regularly appears in APSED documentation (WPRO 2005, 2010, 2016).

In an analysis of ASEAN documentation on infectious diseases, Amaya, Rollet, and Kingah (2015: 239) argue that "the impact of such 'security' framing of a health issue is particularly obvious in the decision of members of ASEAN to enhance their commitments to cooperate in addressing emerging diseases; to develop regional policies to face potential pandemics, notably within the framework of the ASCC Blueprint (2009) and the ASEAN Medium Term Plan on Emerging Infectious Diseases (EID) (2011–2015)." In the 2004, 2006, and 2010 ASEAN Health Ministers Meetings, specific reference is made to the "health emergencies" created by SARS and H5N1 but also endemic diseases including dengue, tuberculosis, malaria, and HIV. Repeated references are made in the 2006 joint statement to the need for "unity" to "protect and prepare" the region during health emergencies. The 2006 statement commits ASEAN states to "develop and implement a regional agreement that institutionalises regional monitoring, reporting and response to outbreaks of communicable diseases, and facilitates the deployment of multinational ASEAN outbreak response teams to assist each other in times of emergencies" (AHMM 2006). The 2010 statement refers at length to the range of "public health threats" the region faces and the intent of health ministers to "task Senior Officials to work out effective regional cooperative arrangements in the prevention, preparedness response to emerging infectious diseases as laid down in the ASEAN Socio-Cultural Community Blueprint 2009–2015" (AHMM 2010).

In the specific material addressing the H5N1 outbreak, such as the 2008 ASEAN Regional Strategy for the Progressive Control and Eradication of Highly Pathogenic Avian Influenza (2008–2010)—published during the virus-sharing crisis—the document states, "HPAI has become endemic and continues to spread in some other countries and, therefore, *remains a threat to the poultry and livestock industry and to public health security in the region and globally*" (ASEAN 2007: 2). In a joint statement with the APT Health Ministers in 2008, there was reference to the "borderless health problems" faced by the region: "We are of the view that in the era of globalisation and trade liberalisation, HIV and AIDS, avian and pandemic influenza, and other emerging infectious diseases continue to *threaten the lives of people in the region*, especially the vulnerable populations, with socio-economic consequences that pose a formidable challenge to ASEAN community building" (APT Health Ministers Meeting 2008). And in the ASEAN Health Ministers' "Call for Action on the Control and Prevention of Dengue" (ASEAN 2011), the statement referred to multilateral alignments in combating disease "threats": "The Asia Pacific Dengue Strategic Plan is in line with the Asia Pacific Strategy for Emerging Diseases (APSED). APSED is a bi-regional strategy endorsed by Member States of the WHO South-East Asia Region and Western Pacific Region, to strengthen national and regional capacities to manage and respond to emerging disease threats including Dengue." A common theme across these statements and blueprints is the alignment of regional health security with regional political leadership and regional cooperation.

However, it remains also true that most of the discussion concerning ASEAN's response to infectious diseases has focused on language and the coordination of events to agitate for funding and shape a collective appreciation of the threat. The domestic mechanisms of response have been largely left to the individual actions of member states with one exception, the Asia Pacific Strategy for Emerging Diseases.

APSED

As the above demonstrates, ASEAN was one of the few regional institutions that consistently and collectively framed emerging infectious disease outbreaks as a threat to regional security. In annual statements, meetings, and blueprints, the membership repeatedly articulated the need to address regional weaknesses in outbreak surveillance and response collectively post-SARS. At the same time as these discussions were taking place within ASEAN, two WHO regional offices within the Asia Pacific region—the Regional Office for the Western Pacific and the South-East Asia Regional Office—proposed a "biregional strategy for strengthening capacity for communicable disease surveillance and response" (WPRO 2005: 5) that was passed by the SEARO and WPRO member states in 2005 (respectively, SEA/RC58/R5 2005 and WPRRC56/R4 2005). The strategy, known as the Asia Pacific Strategy for Emerging Diseases, developed five programs[1] that SEARO and WPRO member states were to implement in order to meet the broader requirements of the revised IHR (2005) and to ensure that national surveillance and response led to "timely and transparent sharing of information" across the two regions (WPRO 2005). When the first phase (2005–2010) of the APSED strategy was reviewed in 2010, it was noted that the ASEAN grouping and its secretariat (which was allowed to attend APSED meetings from 2007) were among the most committed to the early-warning response and surveillance capacity-building projects that were crucial to fulfilling the prompt and transparent reporting function (Heywood and Moussavi 2010: 9). Moreover, this commitment was reflected in the progress both regions had made toward improving surveillance, detection, and response during outbreak events (Chan et al. 2010). ASEAN's engagement in APSED also meant that its member states—half of whom were affected by H5N1 poultry and human outbreaks[2] at the time—had a familiar grouping and secretariat to assist with interpreting reporting obligations to the region and the wider international community. At this stage, there were three layers of institutions that were crucial in shaping ASEAN's engagement with APSED. The first layer was the Health Division under the ASEAN secretariat, which reports to the ASEAN Social-Cultural Community section, which hosts the biannual ASEAN Health Minister Meetings, which seek "political commitment" to a number of technical health issues that require cross-border cooperation (Anonymous 2011c, 2012a). The AHMM produces the ASEAN Health blueprint for medium-term (five-year) planning on health priorities, as well as specific planning and guidelines on responses to individual outbreaks such as H5N1 and dengue (see above). In addition, the AHMM decides on political engagement priorities for health ministries. One key cooperative agreement from the AHMM, inspired by both the SARS outbreak in 2003 and the ongoing H5N1 avian influenza cases in humans and poultry in the region since late 2003–early 2004, was the creation of the APT EID Programme. The ASEAN Expert Group on Communicable Diseases advised the AHMM to establish the APT EID in 2004 in order to achieve technical cooperation for a subset of areas identified as important to fulfilling the broader task of disease detection and reporting. The first task was consultation and cooperation in infectious disease surveillance, which would be approved not just through biannual communiqués by health ministers but also by increased reporting of outbreak events to the APT EID platform (coordinated and operationalized by the Indonesian Ministry of Heath, managed by the ASEAN secretariat and [initially primarily] funded by the Australian Agency for International Development) (Heywood and Moussavi 2010). This platform was dedicated to promoting the "sharing and exchange of timely information on emerging infectious diseases in the region" (APT Health Ministers Meeting 2008).

In addition to the EID surveillance network, the APT EID Programme agreed to a total of four tasks to be developed over three years. Individual states could nominate responsibility for coordinating one of the tasks:

(i) Improvement of institutional capacity of ASEAN to coordinate and manage effective implementation of the program (coordinated by the ASEAN Secretariat);

(ii) Improvement of capacity of the ASEAN Disease Surveillance Network to meet the needs of ASEAN member countries in Emerging Infectious Disease Surveillance, Preparedness and Response (coordinated by Indonesia);

(iii) Improvement of capacity of national and regional laboratories in routine diagnostics, laboratory-based surveillance, preparedness and rapid response (coordinated by Malaysia); and

(iv) Improvement of national and regional capacity in epidemiological surveillance, preparedness, early warning of outbreaks and rapid response to emerging infections (coordinated by Thailand). (ASEAN 2006; AHMM 2006)

There is no evidence here of dissent or muted language concerning reporting responsibility. But the statements above also acknowledged the wider economic costs that H5N1 would have for affected states and constantly stressed the need for international support for ASEAN member states to carry out these programmatic burdens (which were in addition to responding to the H5N1 emergency and rolling out existing health system strengthening programs) (Thomas 2006). ASEAN members, as the agreements illustrate above, saw a direct link between their capacity to improve reporting and the international community's duty to assist them in containing outbreaks and compensating affected industries. Structurally, the APT EID was an additional layer of regional collaboration that strengthened coordination and collaboration within APSED Phase 1.

Furthermore, APT was being helped along with a larger donor push at the time, particularly from the Australian, Canadian, European Union, Japanese, and US donor agencies (Anonymous 2008a). The 2006 ASEAN Health Ministers Statement and the APT Joint Health Ministers statement directly refer to their influence with mention of donors in funding the ASEAN Multi-sectoral Pandemic Preparedness Programme and the APT EID Programme (AHMM 2006; APT Health Ministers Meeting 2008). Likewise, APSED's first phase (2005–2010) was supported financially and diplomatically by the same invested donors, which meant that there was additional interest in making these EID programs "speak" to each other (Anonymous 2010a, 2013a; Australian Government 2017).

A second key subregional institution was the Mekong Basin Disease Surveillance Network among Cambodia, China, Lao PDR, Myanmar, Thailand, and Viet Nam. Since 1999 this informal collaboration of the six countries in the Mekong Basin has met on an annual basis to build "core values of mutual trust, transparency and cooperation" among the health officials in each country. Since 2001, shared knowledge about how to build local capacity to detect disease in border areas, means of sharing outbreak information, and ways of cooperating during an outbreak have been slowly introduced. Two memoranda of understanding (2001 and 2007) have established action plans that guide the work of the MBDS Network in cooperation with the activities of the member states' health ministries (Phommasack et al. 2013).

This subregional framework has been identified in the literature (Kimball et al. 2008) and in personal interviews (Anonymous 2010a, 2010b, 2012c) as has having provided ASEAN states that neighbor each other on the Mekong with a "blame-free" zone in which to communicate disease outbreak events. It was a particular advantage for a majority of new ASEAN member state within the MBDS (Cambodia, Laos, Myanmar, and Viet Nam) to engage in a reporting framework without formal institutional processes. The presence of the overarching international framework to which these member states are bound—the revised International Health Regulations (2005)—served as the impetus for greater reporting cooperation within the MBDS (Phommasack et al. 2013). In addition, during the APSED Phase 1 discussions, the MBDS also served to provide an important example for publicity-wary states on how to share reporting of events without publicly shaming states with differentiated capacity in detection and surveillance (Anonymous 2010a).

Finally, on top of the "thin gruel" (Acharya 2004: 148) of Asian regional institutions are, in the area of health, the WHO WPRO and SEARO. The SEARO membership is 11 countries—Bangladesh, Bhutan, the Democratic Republic of Korea (North Korea), India, Indonesia, the Maldives, Myanmar, Nepal, Sri Lanka, Thailand, and Timor-Leste. The WHO WPRO is a much larger institution, with 37 member countries.[3] SEARO is host to three ASEAN states—two of which have been members of ASEAN since 1967 (Indonesia and Thailand, Myanmar accepted as a member in 1998). The WPRO is host to the remaining six members of ASEAN (Brunei, Cambodia, Laos, Malaysia, Singapore, and Viet Nam).

Unusually, the WPRO and SEARO formed a relationship in early 2005 to develop the first implementation arrangement to address the containment of emerging infectious disease in the region: the Asia Pacific Strategy for Emerging Diseases (Phase 1: 2005–2010; since followed by Phase 2: 2010–2015 and Phase 3: 2015–2020). APSED was described as a framework that would assist member states of both regional offices to adapt and prepare for the core capacities required under the revised IHR (2005) (WPRO 2005).

As noted above, the securitization of infectious disease discourse and corresponding disease response programs within the Asian region—specifically among the APT process—intensified markedly following the SARS outbreak. The swift arrival of H5N1 poultry outbreak after SARS, including poultry-human cases, justified the identification of Southeast Asia as the next epicenter of an influenza pandemic (Jones et al. 2008; WPRO 2010: 12–13). These events, novel disease outbreaks[4] with no known etiology or cure, appeared to justify the choice by those within the WHO to securitize infectious diseases back in the mid-1990s (Davies, Kamradt-Scott, and Rushton 2015: chap. 1). It also appeared to justify the ASEAN secretariat's move toward identifying infectious disease outbreaks as a potential nontraditional security threat (Caballero-Anthony 2008).

It was no doubt this backdrop that led to the APSED project being framed as a "health security" project (Li and Kasai 2011) and to ASEAN member states' comfort with the framework. In 2008, the biannual ASEAN Health Ministers Meeting joint statement referred at length to the activities that ASEAN member states had achieved through their commitment to APSED and their anticipation of continued commitment (note: this statement was made during the height of the virus-sharing disagreement between the WHO and Indonesia):

> We support the Plan of the ASEAN Plus Three EID Programme to develop and implement medium-term and long-term plans to sustain regional cooperation for prevention and control of emerging infectious diseases through multisectoral and integrated approaches in support of International Health Regulation (2005) and Asia Pacific Strategy for Emerging Infectious Diseases (APSED). The Health Ministers agreed that future collaboration will include initiatives to address treatment of emerging infectious diseases. (APT Health Ministers Meeting 2008)

In 2009, the ASEAN secretariat stated at the WPRO regional assembly that the APT EID Programme not only continued to support the implementation of the revised IHR revision and APSED, but the WHO and ASEAN's relationship was deepening because of these structural arrangements:

> Both WHO and ASEAN have value-add in facilitating and coordinating regional follow-up on health development issues of concern. ASEAN-WHO collaboration is based on the comparative advantage of both organizations, and has helped tremendously ASEAN in realizing priorities identified by ASEAN Health Ministers and their senior officials to realize a Healthy ASEAN by 2020. We are pleased to inform you that ASEAN and WHO are now in process of preparing the signing of a new Memorandum of Understanding (MOU) between the two organizations for 2009–2013, to replace the one that was implemented from 1997 to 2007. The new MOU will signify renewed and intensified collaboration between the two organizations. (WPR/RC60/NGO/14)

As will be discussed in the next chapter, APSED facilitated an approach to IHR compliance that was tailored to achieve what was politically feasible and responsive to differentiated capacity (Anonymous 2010l). Given the priority APT EID had dedicated to surveillance and response as early as 2004, the revised

IHR Core Capacity 3 and 4: disease reporting and surveillance, were among the first programs attached to APSED's first phase (after consultation with member states on what was achievable and desirable among most states) (Li and Kasai 2011; Li 2013). It was no coincidence that the prioritization of these two core capacities mimicked the priorities of the first years of the APT EID Programme (Anonymous 2011c).

APSED emerged out of recognition that global health security needed to be responsive to "functional national and regional systems and capacities for managing emerging diseases and acute public health events and emergencies" (Li and Kasai 2011). Crucially, IHR compliance was presented in the APSED model as a capacity-building exercise that would strengthen health systems. The language and program of engagement developed for APSED was, as this chapter has shown, built on the tradition of how ASEAN member states had collectively viewed and pursued regional health security. As the next chapter will demonstrate, APSED did not demand a formal institutional arrangement but instead identified politically feasible priorities, engaged existing regional structures, and kept the terms of membership to the framework flexible to ensure continued buy-in while permitting individual adaption according to health system capacity.

Conclusion

Southeast Asian states have been consistently receptive to the IHR and the need to be IHR compliant. The combination of disease outbreak events and familiarization with the securitization of health and infectious disease discourse created an environment where ASEAN states recognized the threat as shared and understood that collective action was needed to address the threat. The revised IHR contained no extraordinary measures to *compel* shared communication of disease outbreak events, but the H5N1 outbreak, so close to the SARS outbreak, created a different kind of compulsion to cooperate among the ASEAN membership. In a situation where there was such differentiated capacity among ASEAN states and the revised IHR (still) relied on the voluntary compliance of states, the securitization language and approach framework suited the sovereign noninterference model quite well (Heymann 2006). The revised IHR met the sovereign self-interest test for member states committing to a process that would improve performance (particularly if funding was attached). In addition, the securitization discourse would assist with—as chapters 5 and 6 demonstrate—creating shared expectations, even peer pressure, that would push the most reluctant states closer to surveillance and response compliance.

CHAPTER FOUR

Forging Political Support

For many states in Southeast Asia, meeting the revised IHR conditions required quite dramatic changes to legislation and reporting processes within national bureaucracies, and the provision of additional epidemiological training and laboratory capacity. These changes were required just to have the capacity to respond to disease verification requests from the WHO (Baker and Fidler 2006). Southeast Asian states responded to the challenge primarily through a program rolled out as a combined framework between the WHO's WPRO and SEARO offices—the Asia Pacific Strategy for Emerging Diseases. For the first phase of its project implementation, 2005–2010, the program harnessed political support for IHR compliance through two approaches: a focus on "combatting" infectious diseases as a security threat and the development of a regional epistemic community that would drive collaboration on capacity building.

In this chapter, I explore the pursuit of APSED's two-pronged approach in its first phase of implementation, which, alongside sustained engagement with regional governments, sought to promote the normalization of outbreak reporting and shared, collective approaches to outbreak events. I examine the ASEAN secretariat's relationship with APSED and whether this unusual political-technical partnership served to sustain executive-level support for the IHR among the ASEAN membership. Through APSED, ASEAN and the WHO became members of a unique regional network focused on IHR compliance. As this chapter reveals, in the first phase of implementation, APSED's novelty lay in the idea of an approach to IHR compliance tailored to regional needs and sensitive to different health system capacities and different political systems.

The APSED endeavor was deliberately constructed as a "health security" project (Li and Kasai 2011): "In providing a streamlined approach to addressing the *threat of emerging diseases*, APSED has given Member States a powerful tool to coordinate donor funding and to align previously disjointed programme activities towards systematically building strong public health systems" (WPRO 2012: 13; emphasis added). The first phase of APSED involved consultation with member states on regional priorities that supported the promotion of eight core capacities of the recently adopted IHR, but particular attention was given to prioritizing five areas: surveillance and response, laboratory, zoonoses, risk communication, and infection prevention and control. One action that facilitated the realization of these five areas was given particular attention between 2005 and 2010: to "normalize" disease outbreak reporting and, in turn, to attach this performance to strong public health system capacity to conduct detection and reporting. "As well as heading off potential outbreaks, strong surveillance systems can have a widespread impact on the health of a society. Monitoring trends in diseases enables officials to make informed decisions about how to best protect their populations" (WPRO 2010: 16).

In this chapter, I will explore the argument that creating the programmatic objectives of APSED helped support increasing compliance with the IHR in Southeast Asia. It proceeds in three stages. First, the chapter examines the two relevant regional organizations (WPRO and SEARO) attached to WHO headquarters but also decentralized in their budgets, appointment of regional directors, and regional assembly processes. The chapter then turns to how this decentralized structure permitted the development of a unique shared implementation arrangement, the Asia Pacific Strategy for Emerging Diseases (Phase 1: 2005–2010) between WPRO and SEARO. In the third section, the chapter explores the political and financial drivers behind APSED's development during its first phase and studies the outcomes of the 2010 review of APSED's first phase. The analysis of this first phase of APSED reveals two important findings: first, it was not inevitable that APSED would unite a broad selection of diverse member states across two large regions to understand and prepare for the core capacities required under the revised IHR. Second, there were many times during the first phase and in the review of the first phase where there was dissatisfaction and genuine concern about the compliance pull of APSED. Therefore, I am not arguing that APSED is a "perfect" example of cross-regional cooperation, but its creation and continuation was a unique response to the need to adapt a complex, demanding, international framework within a regional setting that enhanced regional cooperation and enabled improved compliance with the IHR.

A Tale of Two Regional Organizations: SEARO and WPRO

In the previous chapter I showed that the securitization of infectious disease discourse and corresponding disease response programs within the Southeast Asian region intensified as a result of the SARS outbreak. The swift onset of the H5N1 poultry outbreak immediately after SARS, including poultry-human cases, supported the increasingly prevalent view that Southeast Asia was the next epicenter of an influenza pandemic (Jones et al. 2008). Between 2005 and 2010, it is no exaggeration that the East Asian region was facing extreme pressure from the aftermath of SARS and the uncertainty around the spread and lethality of H5N1 avian influenza. Among ASEAN states, Indonesia[1] and Viet Nam were the worst-affected states in the region with seasonal H5N1 poultry and human cases. These events, novel disease outbreaks[2] with no known etiology or cure, gave rise to the deliberate securitization of infectious disease to elevate its political status to a regional priority and to dedicate proportional resources to it (see the previous chapter; also Davies, Kamradt-Scott, and Rushton 2015: chap. 3). Investment and development assistance prioritized pandemic preparedness, event-based surveillance networks, desktop simulation exercises, national strategic plans, and antiretroviral stockpiling (Wilsmore et al. 2010).

The adoption of the IHR revisions in 2005 further accelerated states' efforts to appear disease-response ready (the cutoff date for IHR compliance was 2012 for all states, but low-income states could request a delay up to 2014). As chapter 1 has already discussed, responding within a 24–48 hour time frame, as agreed to in 2005, requires a sophisticated communication strategy between local and central health units, rapid disease diagnostic capability (including specimen transfer scheme between location and lab), and a policy process (legislative or regulatory) that allows the IHR focal point (the WHO's verification contact person within the government) to report to the WHO in a timely fashion.

These challenges were magnified by the fragmentation of global health governance in Southeast Asia across two WHO regional organizations: the WHO Western Pacific and South-East Asia regional offices. Three of ASEAN's members are SEARO members (Indonesia, Myanmar, and Thailand); the remaining ASEAN members are WPRO members. SEARO has a membership base of 11 countries; WPRO has 37.[3] At the time of APSED's creation, the SEARO budget had been consistently larger than WPRO's, while its average health performance indicators and health expenditure were significantly lower.[4] However, the total government expenditure on health in 2008 among the Western Pacific membership was (on average) 5.8%, compared to SEARO's 3.8%; and private expenditure in the SEARO region was 58.7%, compared to WPRO's 31.1% (WHO 2017b). Average life expectancy in the Western Pacific region is 75, compared to 65 in SEARO; and the infant mortality rate for children under 1 in SEARO is 45 per 1,000, compared to 18 in the Western Pacific (WHO 2017c).

In sum, these are different offices with different priorities and practices. However, the offices came together to agree on mutual policy, definition, emerging infectious disease response, and IHR implementation in an unusual illustration of institutional readjustment to meet a shared concern. What has been less discussed is why this happened and how it has worked in practice. Below, I introduce how APSED developed out of WHO headquarters' own effort to reform disease outbreak alert and response since the mid-1990s, a reform that has filtered through to inform both state and regional behavior in East Asia and culminated in APSED's creation.

From the outset, there was basic regional consensus on the need to strengthen responses to disease outbreaks—a consensus born of recent experience and concern about the future. Within the regional meetings of SEARO and WPRO to discuss the draft IHR in 2004, some disquiet was expressed about the lack of donor (financial) investment attached to the proposed IHR revisions and, in this vein, about the pressure of balancing the need to dedicate more resources to detection measures for infectious disease with maintaining investment in addressing endemic health problems (both communicable and noncommunicable diseases) already exacting a heavy toll on societies (Davies, Kamradt-Scott, and Rushton 2015: chap. 2). Revisions to the draft IHR were made to accommodate these concerns: reference to a funding mechanism and the creation of a WHA member states–only early-warning disease notification site. A year after these consultations, the revised IHR were passed in 2005. This assent has been interpreted as evidence of the degree to which infectious disease response had been successfully securitized—no state in 2005 spoke *openly* against expanding the IHR coverage, its increased reporting obligations, or the economic investment required to meet the core capacities (Zacher and Keefe 2008: 72–74). Others, however, have been more cautious with their assessment of this assent, suggesting states committed to revisions that were in their interests and in the knowledge there would no repercussions if core capacities were not met (Price-Smith 2009: 154). Where there was dissent, it was mitigated with careful reshaping of concepts and priorities. As Weir and Mykhalovskiy (2010: 56) note, East Asia's *own* framework of IHR implementation took account of these concerns. Here the result was, as noted by those close to APSED's first phase, a top-down approach where states were told what was required and the focus was primarily to meet the region's interests and accommodate "minimum" capacity (Li and Kasai 2011: table 1).

The first material on APSED published by the WPRO and SEARO established an implementation framework that covered both emerging infectious diseases and "other epidemic-prone diseases" specific to the Asia Pacific region (WPRO 2005), suggesting that the two elements are mutually supporting and not in tension with one another. Weir and Mykhalovskiy (2010: 56, 61) argue that this "reconstruction" and expansion of emerging infectious diseases was a distinct reaction, led by the "global South," to a narrower focus on infectious disease supported by the "global North." Some in the global North—Finland, Sweden, Norway, and the Netherlands—however, were as consistent as many African states (and perhaps more so than almost all Asian states) in noting year after year at the Executive Board and WHA sessions that excessive vertical investment in disease preparedness would not address the incapacity problems faced by poor national health systems and gave rise to poor responses to disease outbreaks. In addition to expanding the EID concept to include endemic infectious diseases specific to the region, the second development of the regionalized approach to disease surveillance and response was its relatively quick adoption of WHO's dual themes—securitization of EIDs and coordinated cooperation to implement the IHR. I now consider these developments in more detail.

APSED's Origins

The WHO's reform priorities often include mention of a less region-centric WHO and a more centralized organization (i.e., Gostin et al. 2016; Moon et al. 2015). The Ebola outbreak in West Africa in 2014 amplified these concerns, with commentators (and some in the WHO) assigning blame for the WHO's delayed response to the gravity of the outbreak at the door of the WHO's African regional office (Boseley 2015; Sengupta 2015). Initially, however, the importance of developing regionally tailored pathways to the implementation of the IHR was widely recognized. Regional adaptions of EID core capacities under the IHR were not originally opposed by those from headquarters guiding the IHR revisions, nor did they consider that the global EID focus would suffer from being translated into specific regional strategies (Anonymous 2007a, 2007b, 2008c). At the outset, reference was made to regionally led initiatives in polio surveillance and their contribution to broader disease detection to illustrate the benefit of revised IHR. Therefore, at the time, the creation of a regional adaption of the IHR to reflect regional policy and legal frameworks was not opposed as a novel response to EID. When specifically invited to discuss the adoption of the first phase of APSED, many WHO headquarters officials referred to it as a potential example of "building performance expectations amongst a closer network of member states" (Anonymous 2007a, 2007b). In other words, regional initiatives were seen as positive developments that could drive competition to meet the IHR core capacities.

Within this context, APSED was developed as a bespoke regional road map to guide countries in strengthening their core capacities to meet the IHR revisions (2005). APSED was given substance and direction by the adoption of the IHR revisions in 2005, but it was equally the local product of the region's experience of SARS and H5N1. The region's governments wholly affirmed the IHR revisions in 2005, and most did not attach any reservations to the legal framework.[5] This is remarkable in itself for a region with a history of eschewing international legal obligations (S. Davies 2007). Giorgetti (2012: 1374) has argued that the relatively smooth and rapid adoption of the revised IHR illustrates the possibility for uncontested affirmation by states when the international legal instrument is seen as legitimate, even possibly just and fair. It also, of course, shows that most states viewed the new regulations as supporting their own interests—and, in the case of ASEAN states, interests already framed by the securitization of infectious disease (Calain 2007; Price-Smith 2009: 154). This general acceptance of the IHR by Southeast Asian states gives context to their support for the APSED framework. The IHR met the test of legitimacy and interest. The task of APSED's first phase was to tailor the IHR to a regional road map for states to meet their IHR core capacities (Heywood and Moussavi 2010: 13). However, this was not as simple a proposal as it sounds.

The APSED initiative was the first time that the WPRO and SEARO had sought to develop a health policy document that required all member states to self-report achievements in objectives identified collaboratively to meet IHR core capacity. APSED was not just a geopolitical first but the representation of an important threshold being crossed: regional collaboration to meet individual obligations. The difficulty was going to be choosing the best course of action to meet the rather daunting requirements of IHR core capacity for a diverse group of states that, despite their shared regional membership, ranged across the spectrum when it came to health expenditure, health system capacity, and political regime type. This was going to be a challenge even in subregional contexts like Southeast Asia, with an existing regional institution that has a tradition of seeking coordinated policy among a diverse membership.

APSED—the First Phase

APSED was the outcome of negotiations held in the 55th session of the Regional Committee of the Regional Office for the Western Pacific in 2004 on the provisional item of "Outbreak Response, including Severe Acute Respiratory Syndrome (SARS), Influenza, and revision of the International Health Regulations" (WPR/RC55.5 2004). The committee recommended that then–WPRO director-general Dr. Shigeru Omi develop with SEARO regional director Dr. Samlee Plianbangchang a "biregional strategy for strengthening capacity for communicable disease surveillance and response" (WPR/RC56/7 2005). A year later, the draft Asia Pacific Strategy for Emerging Diseases was presented in both WPRO and SEARO Regional Committees, the same year the IHR revisions were passed (in 2005). WPRO and SEARO officials instrumental in developing APSED stress that the program was always a joint enterprise between the two offices, though many also point to the leadership of Dr. Takeshi Kasai, then-head of Emerging Diseases Surveillance and Response, Division of Health Security and Emergencies at WPRO, who, after the SARS outbreak, was a critical advocate for strengthening regional capacity and, then, for the development and promotion of APSED.

The 2005 APSED report emphasized regional cooperation to assist individual states in meeting the "surveillance, reporting, verification, notification and response capacities" required to implement the revised IHR (WPRO 2005: 3). The report reflected what had been articulated by the WHO secretariat since the mid-1990s: emerging infectious disease is a threat to both developed and developing health systems, and there is a need to combat this threat through coordinated cooperation among states. Of course, what was markedly different in the APSED report was its reference to the region's recent experience of disease threat and the need to achieve regional cooperation to address the threat (WPRO 2005: 5).

Emphasis on regional cooperation was consistently and persistently highlighted in the report: "Countries in the Western Pacific and South-East Asia Regions share significantly large border areas and experience common communicable disease problems such as SARS and avian influenza. There is an urgent need to strengthen biregional collaboration." The benefit of cross-border cooperation is that "networks can play a critical role in improving effective collaboration among partners" (WPRO 2005: 5). Furthermore, the report argued that there are "very few urgent public health risks [that] are solely within the purview of national authorities. The prevention of and response to emerging diseases will need more effective inter-country and inter-regional collabora-tion" (4). It went on to note that SARS and H5N1 demonstrate that "all countries must be prepared" and outlines the specific vulnerability of the Asia Pacific region:

> Many countries are still vulnerable to future disease outbreaks and most coun-tries are still not well prepared for early detection and rapid response to emerging diseases. The importance of strengthening capacities at local levels needs to be recognized, as it is essential for early detection and rapid response to outbreaks ... Therefore, there is an urgent need to develop additional joint activities under the guidance of the strategy in an effort to strengthen national and regional ca-pacities and to reinforce mechanisms to detect, verify, notify and respond rapidly and effectively to emerging diseases and other public health emergencies of na-tional and international concern. (5)

Three important messages come out of the justification for the biregional (WPRO and SEARO) strategy from the report. First, there is *biregional* ac-ceptance of the argument that emerging infectious diseases constitute a secu-rity threat. Though the term "risk" is used in this document in contrast to the "threat" language evoked by the WHO secretariat in the 1990s and 2000s, the referent is the same: emerging infectious diseases affect trade and public health at the national and international level and, in turn, alter the traditional distinc-tion between national and international health (4).

Second, regional cooperation is essential to combat the emerging infectious disease risk effectively. This requires the "development of collaborative net-works at the regional and subregional level for surveillance and response, laboratory, infectious control, and zoonoses" (WPRO 2005: 5). Cooperation is presented as having two roles, collaborative and progressive: collaborative in terms of surveillance, training, and evaluation; progressive in the sense of capacity-building programs to meet the revised IHR core capacity requirements and attract donor funding through direct investment in the framework, private-public partnerships for health financing and knowledge transfer, or both. The relationship here is clear—if states pursue a collective approach to capacity building, they will be in a stronger position to attract donor funding than they would be individually. Indeed, this was the strategy adopted by the region's states affected by H5N1 at the beginning of that outbreak in 2004 and 2005.

Third, the 2005 APSED document (WPRO 2005: 12–15) does not contest the identification of the Asia Pacific as a potential epicenter for future disease outbreaks that may be emerging, reemerging, and epidemic prone. However,

IHR preparedness is presented as an opportunity to address the "*differences* between the countries in their current level of preparedness for emerging diseases, and therefore their capacity strengthening needs . . . by generic recommendations for adaption to the local situation" (12; emphasis added). APSED focused on collaboration to establish a level health playing field in the region. Awareness of the discrepancies across public health systems is repeatedly referred to in the 2005 APSED document (3, 5, 18–19). If local capacity is not strengthened, then states will not be able to meet core IHR requirement for surveillance and response (5). As such, the emphasis in APSED was to improve "health protection" in the Asia Pacific region through the achievement of five objectives (of equal importance but adaptable to local priorities regarding implementation):

1. Objective 1—reduce the risk of emerging diseases
2. Objective 2—strengthen early detection of outbreaks of emerging diseases
3. Objective 3—strengthen early response to emerging diseases
4. Objective 4—strengthen preparedness for emerging diseases
5. Objective 5—develop sustainable technical collaboration within the Asia Pacific Region

An Asia Pacific Technical Advisory Group for Emerging Infectious Diseases (TAG EID) was established and first met in July 2006. As a "track two" (nonofficial) body, its role was to advise states on the specific steps that were required. Beyond this, the management structure of APSED was primarily composed of a modest secretariat, with communicable disease unit representations from SEARO and WPRO, and a Partners' Forum whose membership primarily consisted of donors, multilateral organizations, UN agencies, intergovernmental and nongovernmental organizations, professional associations, and subregional networks. The TAG EID sat underneath the secretariat and Partners' Forum (both of which fed into an executive function for managing the strategy—primarily led by the secretariat) and was responsible to the Executive Committee (not the secretariat or, note, the Partners' Forum). TAG was to oversee planning and implementation of the strategy, provide technical support, monitor progress, advise of implementation in technically related matters and policy, convene working groups for programs, identify external advisers, advise the Partners' Forum and keep them informed, and review and revise the strategy. As an informal network, membership varied over time, with observers included from key United Nations agencies and intergovernmental technical partners from the region (e.g., the ASEAN secretariat and South Asian Association for Regional Cooperation secretariat were recorded in minutes as attending from 2007) (WPRO 2005: 39–40).

At its first meeting, TAG advised that states should adopt an APSED work plan, with "explicit links to the IHR (2005), to develop a checklist for countries to measure performance against the work plan, to identify the appropriate audit tools and baseline capacities for self-assessment," and to evaluate laboratory capacity and capability in all countries to determine diagnostic capacity for emerging infectious diseases. From the outset, TAG argued that APSED should be understood as a long-term project. For example, it was noted in the 2006 TAG that if a few countries could complete the five objectives within five years, this would represent the completion of "stage one" of a longer-term strategy and create impetus for further phases of work (WPRO-SEARO 2006: 20). Indeed, this view has come to pass with APSED having just confirmed its third-phase framework (2015–2020).

The first stage of APSED was directed at three levels: first, establishing biregional cooperation and networking; second, promoting subregional collaboration; and, third, capacity building in communicable disease surveillance and response at the national level. APSED was to cover all EIDs, but, again reflective of its adaption to regional needs, the priority in the first phase was to implement emergency arrangements for "avian and pandemic influenza as soon as possible" (WPRO-SEARO 2006: 20). Advocacy for a strategy that took into account regional needs and priorities was based on the argument that "there is a window of opportunity to fundamentally strengthen national and international public health systems for alert and response to emerging infectious diseases using the resources made available for the control of avian influenza and pandemic preparedness activities" (7). Essentially, donor investment and political momentum in response to the highly publicized avian influenza outbreak made this an opportune time to use pandemic preparedness as the funding base for developing and testing early warning and response (19, 21, 22).

Developing a program from the five APSED objectives outlined for the first phase (above), and taking into account the donor and political interest at the time, five program areas were identified to form the APSED work plan for 2005 to 2010:

1. Surveillance and response
2. Laboratory development
3. Infection control

4. Zoonoses

5. Risk communication

The sixth program area—the WHO's regional function and activities—was not discussed by the time of the 2006 TAG EID. This decision, it appears, resulted from the simple realization that the first five program areas would all require WHO cooperation at the country, regional, and headquarters level (Anonymous 2008d).

In its 2006 meeting, TAG advised that the APSED work plan should be used as the "framework and guidance for countries and partners to meet the commitments of the IHR (2005)." It further argued that implementing this work plan would be expected for the states under APSED to meet the surveillance and response requirement of the IHR (2005) (WPRO-SEARO 2006: 22). In 2007, feedback started to come in from the assessment tasks adopted on the advice of the 2006 TAG. It should be noted that this "airing" at a biregional forum of how member states were progressing individually and collectively meeting the five APSED program areas was novel.[6]

Worried about potential slippage on the timetable for implementation, in 2006 TAG called for greater high-level political commitment to support ministries of health in resourcing for the five APSED programs (WPRO-SEARO 2006: 22). Nonetheless, in 2007, TAG EID reported that political commitment and resources were still insufficient and that this posed an impediment to achieving successful outcomes in the five program areas (WPRO-SEARO 2007: 1). A presentation from the Communicable Disease Surveillance and Response (CSR) unit within SEARO, reported the "main challenges in implementation include technical strengthening of core capacities within countries, mobilization of resources and national political commitment to rapidly share information and material, and political support for inter-country collaboration" (5). From analyzing the TAG discussion records in 2007, it seems that the primary concern was whether states would be transparent with their disease reporting and, in turn, whether there was sufficient political commitment to meet all the goals (5, 15, 21). On the matter of disease reporting, for example, it was noted that WHO headquarters, not regional offices, should lead the majority of disease verification requests, especially those that require risk assessment in establishing whether they posed a "public health emergency of international concern" (9). Was this a reminder or an admonishment?

Interviews with those present at TAG meetings put forward different opinions on this discussion from the 2007 TAG. Some thought it was delivered as a gentle reminder to some states that they could communicate in private to regional offices but that they also needed to demonstrate their compliance to the IHR by engaging in public reporting (Anonymous 2008d, 2012b). The concern was that APSED had progressed so well that states were far more comfortable with internal and private regional reporting processes than they were with more public reporting. Others believed that this advice came from those allied with WHO headquarters who wanted to assert the importance of verification to *them* and their event management system rather than through the informal channels used in regional offices (phone calls and individual emails between Ministry of Health offices and WPRO or SEARO officials) (Anonymous 2008c, 2010m).

Despite the agreement on APSED's first-phase work plan, the two regions maintained different interpretations of the APSED program for pursuing the biregional strategy. At the annual TAGs, the suggested practice from 2006 was for each region to present information about its collective performance against the five APSED program areas. Individual states could also present their progress against the five program areas. Turning to the implementation status of recommendations from the 2006 APSED TAG meeting—SEARO's regional adviser on CSR, Dr. Khanchit Limpakarnjanarat—presented a story of progress. To some observers in TAG, presenting a story of progress at this stage was worrying because there was doubt that all states were progressing, and couching it in these terms would make it harder for "honest" feedback (Anonymous 2008c, 2010o). Others, however, were not concerned, noting there was a difference between what was recorded and what was discussed in breakout sessions (Anonymous 2010a).

In July 2006 a ministerial delegation had passed the Delhi Declaration at a SEARO-convened conference on addressing control efforts of AI. The conference hosted both health and agriculture ministers from Afghanistan, Bangladesh, Bhutan, China, India, Indonesia, the Maldives, Myanmar, Nepal, Sri Lanka, and Thailand. They agreed on the need for implementing surveillance and response capacities at the national and regional levels to reduce the public health threat posed by AI or any other pandemic outbreak (SEARO n.d.: 3).[7] Limpakarnjanarat noted that this political engagement via APSED enabled the creation of CSR subunits in New Delhi and Bangkok to "coordinate IHR, APSED and AI activities, via strengthening of the regional reference laboratory capacities and the constitution of a task force for research on AI" (WPRO-SEARO 2007: 27). SEARO further "supported" a number of outbreak investigations, including in relation to AI outbreaks in Indonesia, Myanmar, and Bangladesh;

chikungunya fever in India and Maldives; and dengue fever in Nepal (5). Although dealing with these emergencies had led to "some delays in APSED implementation" (33), Limpakarnjanarat argued that, through these efforts, SEARO had made significant progress in four areas: (1) implementation of IHR (2005) had been advanced through country assessments and a road map for development of national plans, with a checklist for member states to assess their public health and veterinary laboratory capacity; (2) SEARO was developing a regional strategy for training in field epidemiology and rapid response teams, and developing guidelines on disease surveillance and outbreak response, specifically to AI; (3) a regional framework and meeting was in progress for prevention and control of zoonoses diseases; and (4) "consolidating coordination through biregional planning will be needed in the next phase of APSED implementation" (27–28).

The WPRO report, in contrast, was less glowing. Dr. Kasai, regional adviser for CSR for WPRO and Limpakarnjanarat's WPRO equivalent, presented in his overview that progress had been made from 2006 with the formation of working groups for most of the program areas and the start of national assessments of core capacity. However, he identified two areas as possible concerns, where progress was stymied by "human resource constraints": risk communication and infection control. Perhaps in reference to the general TAG discussion on the role of regional offices and WHO headquarters regarding disease verification over the previous year, Kasai argued that exercises and assessments had been devoted to improve regional performance in these areas (WPRO-SEARO 2007: 9). Kasai noted, however, at the conclusion of the session on APSED's work plan that while the five program areas were articulated as "the five pillars of APSED implementation," four sub–working group meetings had not yet been held to establish minimum requirements for program implementation (only surveillance and response—Objective 1—had held its first sub–working group) (26, 28).

WPRO's progress report, presented by Kasai, summarized five areas of work: (1) WPRO had endorsed TAG's first recommendations, and these were now being implemented as a "critical framework and tool for countries to meet commitments in the prevention and control of communicable diseases." (2) A sub–working group meeting on surveillance and response had been established to develop "APSED minimum standards for surveillance and response," and similar sub–working groups were planned for four other program areas. The subgroup membership consisted of a TAG member, a representative from IHR core capacities working group based in WHO Lyon, and officers from WHO country offices and the regional office. (3) An APSED Baseline Data Collection

Checklist was developed that covered the five program areas for country assessments in the Western Pacific region. Furthermore, the assessment was tailored to six countries with the greatest need (these countries had volunteered for this program): Cambodia, Lao PDR, Mongolia, Papua New Guinea, the Philippines, and Viet Nam. (4) The WPRO had developed an APSED sub-work plan for strengthening regional outbreak alert and response capacities that would support regional partnerships in the GOARN, as well as a sub–work plan for strengthening laboratory biosafety. And, finally, (5) the WPRO was seeking to promote human resource development in all of the five program areas to reflect "long-term resourcing at all levels involved in implementation" (WPRO-SEARO 2007: 28–29).

Arguably, the WPRO was more critical than SEARO in identifying the benchmarks to be met within each of the five APSED program pillars—from seeking Regional Committee approval, to creating an APSED Baseline Data Collection Checklist, targeting member states in greatest need of APSED work plans, and reporting shortfalls in implementing the programs—from human resource capacity to a lack of clear implementation strategy for the risk communication program.

In articulating the WPRO's engagement with the five program areas, Kasai also noted that the WPRO had, like SEARO, devoted "advocacy activities to increase political support for APSED" over 2006–2007. Reference to political support for APSED had particular weight to it at this TAG: the ASEAN secretariat had been invited to the proceedings, and its participation would continue from 2007, building the organization into the region's epistemic networks. The decision to include ASEAN in the annual TAG appears to have been the culmination of numerous factors occurring at the same time.

First, it appears that the combined diplomacy of donors and the ASEAN secretariat made the case for the participation of this regional organization in the APSED program. Two particularly strong donor voices were APSED and APT EID donors and WPRO members Australia and Japan, along with officials from within the ASEAN secretariat. The Australian government had been investing in the APT EID Phase 2 (2006–2009), as had the Japanese government (another WPRO member) in APT Phase 1 (2003–2006).

As APSED donors in the first phase, Australia and Japan were important allies for promoting ASEAN's inclusion. In the years that followed, the United States, Canada, and the European Union funded models on pandemic preparedness and global health security that all came to include ASEAN with WPRO and SEARO events (Anonymous 2011d; GHSA 2016; Wilsmore et al.

2010). Why was it important to include ASEAN, given that the combined WPRO and SEARO strategy already included all ASEAN members? Different views were put forward to this question in interviews.

A senior ASEAN official, for example, noted that in prior discussions with the WPRO and SEARO, it was suggested that including the ASEAN secretariat within APSED's deliberations would significantly elevate the level of prioritization given to APSED by Southeast Asian governments (Anonymous 2011c). Did this indicate a concern that APSED was not being taken seriously by some ASEAN members? There are multiple views on the necessity for the ASEAN institution to be identified as a "third partner" to APSED. One view, from interviews with ASEAN secretariat and WHO officials, was that there was growing regional concern about some ASEAN countries continually resisting any external involvement—namely Myanmar and Laos. Neither SEARO nor the WPRO had a political relationship with the executive leadership of both countries. The one institution that did was ASEAN (Anonymous 2008b, 2010a). The preference was to establish a relationship, through a regional "peacetime operation," rather than having to face an emergency when the outbreak and politics could be difficult to contain (Anonymous 2013a). This is where recognition of need for ASEAN's presence was identified.

Another view put forward in interviews was that states such as Indonesia (and Thailand to a lesser extent) were part of SEARO but also wanted to be part of the WPRO discussions. The way to achieve this was to include ASEAN as a member of APSED, which would permit attendance at WPRO events that were not badged as biregional (Anonymous 2008a, 2008c, 2010m). These sources also suggested that Indonesia's close aid relationship with Australia (which is a WPRO member) facilitated this arrangement.

Finally, there was interest from ASEAN itself to highlight the role it was playing in developing capacity-building projects through the APT EID Programme. It was known that some ASEAN states consulted each other informally and were genuinely attempting to build capacity outside of the WHO structure through the APT EID Programme and the Mekong Basin Disease Surveillance Network. Including the ASEAN secretariat into APSED was a tactical move to ensure everyone was on "the same page" (Anonymous 2010a, 2010l, 2010o, 2012a).

As mentioned already, the APSED five program areas were also directly relevant to the objectives being formulated under the APT EID Programme. The ASEAN secretariat was charged with responsibility for rolling out 12 projects for APT EID Phase 2, all of which had been determined after high-level consultations with the Australian government in 2007 and formally adopted by the APT senior health officials and the ASEAN Expert Group on Communicable Diseases later in the year (ASEAN 2014, 2012a, 2012b; UNSIC 2011). One of the important outcomes was a protocol for communication and information sharing, with reporting obligations that pertained to diseases that fell under the IHR (2005) but also diseases under routine surveillance in the region—like dengue, malaria, HIV, tuberculosis, and rabies. Projects within this protocol included the promotion of sharing outbreak event information through a secure website for members (the Indonesia Ministry of Health manages the site), Malaysia's provision of advice and consultation on laboratory-based surveillance information to assist with verification, and Thailand's leadership in fieldwork epidemiology training. To support these activities, it was agreed that partners would also participate in exercises in laboratory training, detection and surveillance, risk communication, familiarization with the IHR, and opportunities for regular communication among focal points.

APSED was therefore identified as providing a further opportunity to expand and familiarize the networks and partnerships sustaining the APT EID strategic plan. From 2007 ASEAN's increased presence in APSED functions increased technical commitment. It facilitated expertise in the form of an ASEAN Expert Group to assist with localization of the five APSED programs, and there were a small number of staff transfer and exchanges between the ASEAN secretariat and WPRO (in particular). More crucially, ASEAN's inclusion brought political support and engagement. ASEAN commitment delivered the approval and engagement of Health Ministers from 10 member states, plus the ministerial engagement of the Plus Three states (China, Japan, and South Korea) and the engagement of donor states' health *and* foreign affairs ministries. Furthermore, given ASEAN's membership spread across SEARO and WPRO membership, the political engagement of ASEAN went some way toward stemming the aforementioned risks of bifurcation between SEARO and WPRO (Anonymous 2011c). There were now 10 states (plus 3) that had a political allegiance that preexisted APSED and was greater than divisions between SEARO and the WPRO.

Finally, there was also the individual factor. Kasai and Limpakarnjanarat were, in hindsight, well placed in their roles as directors of Communicable Disease (at the time) for the WPRO and SEARO, respectively. Both had experience operating within the ASEAN framework. As a Thai national, Limpakarnjanarat was familiar with the diplomatic significance that member states attached to the regional organization, ASEAN. Kasai is a Japanese national but had a long history of working in the Southeast Asian region and was familiar with the diplomatic practice of ASEAN.

However, despite donor, institutional, and individual champions, divisions between SEARO and the WPRO were perhaps the uppermost concern during the first phase. SEARO members in 2007, in contrast to WPRO members, appeared less prepared for pandemic influenza outbreak containment strategies, and, overall, these member states had achieved less progress in meeting core IHR requirements (WPRO-SEARO 2007: 11–12). A SEARO communicable disease official, Dr. Narain, argued that, in SEARO countries, responding to avian influenza was the priority, but so too was responding to their high cases of drug-resistant tuberculosis and vector-borne diseases experienced at the same time (4–5). This was an argument presented by one SEARO official to explain, even defend, discrepancies in implementation and compliance between the regions. There are two ways of interpreting this moment. The first, more positive, is that in spite of APSED being a new technical and political program, only a year later states were willing to openly report their progress (or lack thereof) and engage in discussions directed toward improving performance. The second, more negative, view is that comparing implementation progress highlighted sharp differences among states with vastly different health capacities.

SEARO had no member states with high income and above-average life expectancy. Only 5 out of the 11 SEARO member countries met "most of the criteria" in the initial desk review of existing IHR core capacity. In general, SEARO's own capacity was quite weak, with an "urgent need to build national capacities in endemic alert and response, including cross-border and inter-country surveillance and response activities," that required greater political mobilization among political leadership of SEARO countries. This is not to say that the WPRO was not experiencing difficulties with some of its members being able to achieve minimum capacity by 2010, but the WPRO's desk review had found that its implementation framework would be easier to progress and assess than SEARO's, at least in the earliest stage. It had a number of states that could implement the IHR core capacity criteria relatively quickly and efficiently. This resource ease permitted, for example, the WPRO to identify six states (Cambodia, Lao PDR, Mongolia, Papua New Guinea, the Philippines, and Viet Nam) in which it could devote additional resources and attention in the first phase to assist with core capacity implementation, while in SEARO not one state had reported to the regional office over 2006–2007 for such assistance and not one SEARO member had yet fulfilled all the core capacity criteria for the revised IHR (WPRO-SEARO 2007: 12).

Differences in membership capacity and engagement with their regional office was further reflected in how the regional offices assumed responsibilities for APSED when it was their year to host the TAG. The 2010 review of APSED's first phase noted that, with the annual TAG meeting rotation between the WPRO and SEARO, different styles affected the cooperation and coordination practices for that year:

> The organisation of the meeting, including decisions as to who participates, varies depending on which region is taking responsibility for its organisation. WPRO brings all stakeholders—Member States, donor agencies, technical experts—together, thus facilitating interaction between all parties. Conversely, SEARO separates these groups, and in doing so, limits the amount of interaction that can potentially occur between each of the groups. (Heywood and Moussavi 2010: 16)

The same report went on to note, however, that "prior to APSED there were no formal bi-regional collaboration activities" and that one of the "most significant benefit to this bi-regional approach is that it allows countries to work across borders, eliminating the false separation that is imposed by the WHO regional composition. Close neighbours can also share the same vision and framework even if they are at different stages of developing capacity. They are using the same language, working towards the same goal" (18).

The novelty of the biregional framework and its expectation of open disclosure on the progress of implementation, in an environment where there were different capacities and resources (not to mention political rivalries), carried high expectations. Given this, it is perhaps not surprising that opportunities were sought for pushback. For example, a common critique in the 2007 TAG, hinted at above with the SEARO report, was that APSED placed too much emphasis on strengthening early response to emerging diseases at the expense of other health concerns. One (anonymous) TAG member suggested that some programs, particularly detection and response, received more attention than "equally important" APSED programs: "Strengthening the early response to emergency diseases (APSED Objective 3) had received considerable attention while other programme areas have been neglected" (WPRO-SEARO 2007: 26). This was a common concern heard by those working in TAG and in close proximity to low-income Health Ministry departments that felt the pressure of

APSED as another resourcing burden. It would not be an exaggeration to stress that 2007 was a make-or-break time for the future of APSED.

In July 2008, the APSED TAG met for its third annual meeting to assess annual progress of APSED. Three years had passed since APSED was introduced, and progress was reported, with more than half the countries completing assessments of national surveillance and response systems (25 out of 46 member states), and the same number had drafted national plans to develop core capacities required under the IHR (2005). The WPRO countries identified in 2007 as requiring priority action—Cambodia, Lao PDR, Mongolia, Papua New Guinea, the Philippines, and Viet Nam—had drafted national plans to address their shortfalls within each of the five APSED programs. Furthermore, six SEARO members—Bangladesh, Indonesia, India, Myanmar, Sri Lanka, and Thailand—had agreed at the end of 2007 to "strengthen rapid response capacity at country level through training of national and provincial rapid response teams" (WPRO-SEARO 2008: 2). Sri Lanka also volunteered as the first SEARO country to be evaluated for progress in meeting the five program areas as part of the 2008 midterm review of APSED implementation (Lao PDR was nominated as the WPRO country) (5). The engagement of countries—some previously regarded as distant from the strategy (e.g., Laos and Myanmar) bolstered enthusiasm. There was also more effort devoted to create one story to mobilize WPRO and SEARO states to work together.

The 2008 TAG reported some progress in program areas other than outbreak detection, with training and evaluations done in laboratory diagnostic and biosafety capacity, zoonoses collaboration mechanisms, infection control, and risk communication training. Crucially, implementation of activities under each APSED program area was noted to vary, with risk communication now being the one marked as "behind schedule." The overall assessment of APSED's progress in 2008 was strikingly honest and ambitious: "The [bi]region was not close to achieving the regional goal of national core capacity development by 2010" (WPRO-SEARO 2008: 3). But to keep all states engaged, the 2008–2009 work plan, like the 2007 plan, did not demand massive expectations from member states—the language used was the introduction of "minimum systems and functional areas" in the capability checklist for each program area in each country (4).

Of course, the process of tracking the progress of APSED implementation was crucial to understand its impact at national level. In June 2008, both SEARO and the WPRO conducted the midterm review of one member state from each region—Lao PDR (WPRO) and Sri Lanka (SEARO)—to assess the implementation progress of APSED. However, SEARO and the WPRO had different positions on reporting and assessments. Separate assessment tools were used for measuring implementation: for Laos the APSED implementation monitoring tool was a WPRO checklist; and, for Sri Lanka, SEARO developed its own assessment tool, and the assessment was self-reported (WPRO-SEARO 2008: 6). From its inception, APSED—as with the revised IHR—requires states to map their national capacity, resources, and gaps, and then regional offices determine how the monitoring and evaluation should be conducted by states to self-measure their progress. In 2010, the APSED review noted that this reliance on self-measurement for capacity, performance, and implementation was a mixed bag and led to "documentation of some deliverables of the program, including those underpinning the APSED approach, [to be] considered weak" (Heywood and Moussavi 2010: 15). Some effort had gone into the 2008 meeting to progress honest self-assessment since the 2007 TAG meeting, and while SEARO and the WPRO were using the same framework they were moving in different directions regarding their assessment and envisioned outcomes.

In 2008—and up to the review of APSED's first phase in 2010—TAG progressed with open communication on states reporting their progress according to the original APSED work plan. It was annually noted that TAG's primary responsibility was to chart progress and monitor achievements under the five program areas, and these assessments needed to be "based against established milestones of the WHO APSED workplan" (WPRO-SEARO 2007: 33). The review of APSED's first phase found that while a forum for engagement and sharing experiences in developing capacity had been vital, progressing an understanding of what APSED milestones looked like, and how APSED could assist states with IHR capacity building, was quite different in perception and style across SEARO and the WPRO. In 2008 and 2009, "significant effort" was directed at a strengthened monitoring and evaluation approach with introduction of a "Common Indicator Assessment" (Heywood and Moussavi 2010: 34).

APSED provided a framework that filled the vacuum between what countries could manage and what they had to achieve to be IHR compliant: "Countries have demonstrated that the approach that APSED proposes for building capacity—working with partners, utilising networks—is being embraced and does improve capacity . . . Networks were being used" (Heywood and Moussavi 2010: 43). However, the different methods of organization and engagement by the two regional offices alongside different preferences for monitoring and evaluation limited, at the end of first phase, opportunities for "regional/country comparisons and ultimately assessment of the overall effectiveness of APSED"

(18). Concern with the lack of a "comprehensive biregional picture of APSED progress," as requested in the 2007 TAG by a TAG adviser, was not achieved until just prior to the 2010 review. Even then, the review noted, a comparative measurement of progress across the two regions remained APSED's primary impediment (Heywood and Moussavi 2010).

Regional offices may have had doubts or concerns about states conducting self-reports of progress against the five program areas, but there was also no way of contesting states' individual account of performance in meeting the five programs without direct confrontation. To have pushed for external reporting of national performance would have raised concerns and diminished trust in the progress made to date. One WPRO official, close to the APSED framework, noted the diplomatic difficulties in the first phase but attributed them mostly to the culture of SEARO (unsurprisingly!), arguing that most of its membership would not freely discuss performance limitations in the same way that WPRO members would. An epidemiologist stationed within SEARO confirmed this view, noting that SEARO as an institution was not comfortable with admitting limitations or publishing member state progress—the organization was institutionally set up to meet member states' desire to be presented as performing well and efficiently. In fairness, there was also the fact that the IHR reporting requirements (to headquarters) were being introduced from 2010 and not beforehand. While the APSED framework could assist states' understanding of how they were to meet the reporting expectation, the IHR were the instrument that carried reporting obligations, not APSED.

The first phase of APSED was described by a number of people working within it as an opportunity for the region to better understand the IHR and develop meaningful and carefully tailored work plans for their implementation. If we understand the IHR as a normative process, this first phase was one of normative engagement and socialization (Davies, Kamradt-Scott, and Rushton 2015). APSED promoted discussion between states on how much capacity-building progress needed to be achieved, for national-level technical experts and bureaucrats to share experiences of political discussions within ministries of health, and to build an informal network among IHR National Focal Points to discuss their job in detecting and reporting outbreak messages to regional offices and WHO headquarters. This assessment was supported by a key architect of APSED, who described the first phase as being primarily about preparedness: "It was a tool, to prepare states for [IHR] core capacity [reporting]." The same individual went on to note that the first phase of APSED allowed "states to realize what they need to do to be ready. It will only take one or two states to put everyone at risk and this may still be the case. It wasn't until 2005 that everyone realized having a plan in place would not be enough. TAG realized there would need to be a means to execute it. States needed to be on task with readiness, event notification, and monitoring" (Anonymous 2010m).

How did APSED then manage the politics of its membership? As the APSED review noted, despite TAG's emphasis on technical performance, political cooperation was vital to APSED's success (Heywood and Moussavi 2010: 9). As I examine in more detail below, the review noted that one political impediment to cooperation was continued "political sensitivities to sharing information about outbreaks, and this affects the extent to which some countries will involve themselves with networks. Linked to this is also variable commitment to cross-border cooperation" (17). Crucially, APSED's first phase was judged to be a capacity-building exercise and that "takes time, and significant motivation and energy has been generated in countries to work toward fully implementing IHR requirements. It would be premature for support to this activity to cease in view of such [overall] energy and commitment" (44).

During its first phase APSED was not without difficulties. There were significant differences between the two regional offices in their emphasis on reform, capacity building, and assessment. The process of engagement was technical and top-down, making little use of established political relationships in the region. The expectation of commitment to APSED as distinct or complementary to the IHR revisions was unclear, and adding the APSED layer potentially risked the region's understanding of the IHR implementation process. The focus was on attracting countries to participate and to engage, and this was done by emphasizing minimum capacity and reporting expectations. The organization around the five APSED programs (to be delivered in the first phase) was slow and uneven—with surveillance and response well ahead in implementation, compared to the other four programs. At the same time, APSED progressed a discussion about IHR implementation that was tailored to regional experience and regional needs; the focus was on capacity and linking broader endemic infectious disease concerns to the narrow pandemic focus of IHR implementation (at the time). The first phase of APSED created annual opportunities for epistemic communities to meet and hold frank and informal interaction among public health officials, universities, laboratories, and WHO officials. The inclusion of ASEAN and APT provided political commitment to the APSED framework and added another layer of institutional investment in the biregional approach. APSED was treated as an investment by donor states, and this added to the impression that while the IHR had no funding mechanism, donor states were treating the revisions with seriousness in *this* region. Most importantly, the APSED framework provided a mechanism by which to engage with the norms introduced by the IHR revisions—the duty to report, the duty to respond, the duty to contain. ASEAN states, by virtue of the effort to include the ASEAN secretariat in the APSED framework, were being asked to navigate a pathway to implementation that complemented sovereignty (capacity building) but also challenged the norm of noninterference (shared reports of disease outbreak events). The definition of an ASEAN member state entitled to noninterference was changing—it needed to be able to secure the health of its citizens *and* its region (Caballero-Anthony 2014). This does not mean all ASEAN states were IHR compliant by the end of 2010, but emphasis on continued contact and the creation of regional institutional layers around the IHR revisions created a sense of regional obligation. From 2005, the adoption of the IHR and the presence of APSED, combined with the plan of action under the APT EID, made it increasingly difficult for even the most recalcitrant political regime to openly reject its obligation to detect and report disease outbreak events.

Review of APSED's First Phase

The first phase of APSED had three goals reflected across five program areas it identified as possible within a five-year time frame: increased biregional cooperation and network collaboration in disease reporting and response, subregional collaboration and capacity building in communicable disease surveillance, and political engagement in capacity building and response at the national level. The five program areas prioritized for these goals in the first phase of the APSED program were surveillance and response, laboratory development, infection control, zoonoses, and risk communication.

During APSED's first phase (2005–2010), consensus was strong in that improving individual state performance in the detection, response, and verification of disease outbreaks was consistently advanced to encourage biregional cooperation, build health system capacity, and encourage political engagement. Improving state-level performance in alerting neighbors and the broader international community to disease outbreaks was consistently viewed as the "first line of defense" in disease containment, and APSED devoted significant resources to encourage changes in reporting behavior among states, that is, increasing transparency and normalizing requests for assistance (Coker et al. 2011; Li 2013).

The 2010 review of APSED's performance was primarily based on an analysis of states' self-reported assessments over the APSED phase; interviews with stakeholders in the WHO regional offices; review of the Common Indicator Assessments of the six states that self-indicated a high level of need in 2007 (Cambodia, Laos, Mongolia, Philippines, Papua New Guinea, and Viet Nam); and visits and assessments of Indonesia, Sri Lanka, and Palau (which had individually self-nominated for specific areas of program implementation in the first phase). The review noted that while the countries included in the report had not achieved all the APSED or IHR core capacity benchmarks, there was strong support within these countries for APSED continuing based on state-level feedback that their performance had improved and that the APSED framework was relevant to strengthening their health system capacity (Heywood and Moussavi 2010: 31). In fact, the only area that lacked consistent progress across the region was risk communication, but the review could not detect any "serious attempt to understand why" (27). The review also uncovered "varying degrees" of implementation and participation, with specificity of implementation and participation across the regions (with the exception of the five countries reviewed) being somewhat scant and quite generalized in summary discussions.

APSED sought to specifically address regional needs to improve general disease outbreak response capacity with a view to progressing IHR core capacity requirements (Heywood and Moussavi 2010: 9). This was a midlevel intervention between the state and headquarters by regional offices to promote a regional understanding of what needed to be prioritized in the revised IHR. While, since the mid-1990s, WHO headquarters had sought to normalize alert and response and to promote the use of surveillance networks that engage state and non-state partners, there had been little adoption of these practices in the Asia Pacific region. As mentioned already in the previous chapter, two events that galvanized receptiveness toward WHO regional-level engagement with infectious disease response and containment were the SARS outbreak and H5N1. These events have been identified as the trigger for regional awareness of the need for the IHR revisions (Anonymous 2008c). The broader Asian region[8] was keenly aware of its vulnerability to criticism about state-level institutional failure post–SARS and H5N1. The decision to collaborate regionally was not the only option on the table. Indeed, the 2010 review of APSED was driven in part by a desire to question whether funding should continue (Anonymous 2011c). APSED, as well as APT EID, was to be the promotion of a "common vision approach to EID" while strengthening "health systems and program areas to respond to EID" (Anonymous 2008c, 2011c). The possibility of new financial resources being made available to states, from donors such as Australia, Japan, the EU, Canada, and the United States, to create local capacity through attachment to the APSED five program areas was also a strong incentive for state engagement. Collaborative projects across states and regions did accrue higher investment in the immediate aftermath of the IHR revisions, even if they proved more difficult to measure and manage progress (i.e., Wilsmore et al. 2010).

There was also a concerted effort within the APSED framework and the technical discussions it facilitated—emphasized and repeated in the TAG documents as the years went by—to develop response capacity not just for potential disease outbreaks but to address the endemic diseases already straining individual states' health systems (Anonymous 2008c), that is, to tailor the global health security agenda to better fit pressing regional needs. The APSED framework accommodated the fact that Southeast Asian governments had to contend with the dual risk of emerging infectious diseases (Nipah in 1998, SARS in 2003, and H5N1 in both 1997 and 2004) as well as epidemic-prone diseases (malaria, dengue, and Japanese encephalitis). Moreover, those promoting APSED seemed to not only accept this reality but exploit its potential. One Ministry of Health official from one of the countries that reported its Common Indicator Assessment results, and the recipient of a World Bank pandemic prevention grant, informed the author that the state's pandemic influenza preparedness grant funded a laboratory that primarily serves the community to test Japanese encephalitis and TB (Anonymous 2010e). They did not document this activity because they did not want to jeopardize future funding, but these types of practices were recounted to the author across the region in interviews during the first five years of APSED. Even World Bank officials in the region freely acknowledged that they knew this regularly occurred, and this acceptance of informal crossover between vertical and horizontal health funding was "not a concern" as long as donors got to see the laboratory and confirmed the PCR tests (for influenza) could be done if called upon (Anonymous 2010d).

Of course, most of the time such liberal use of funds was not possible, but it does point to why some individuals connected to APSED may have been reluctant to be too demanding of progress indicators. Financial and political momentum on pandemic influenza preparedness was at an all-time high pre–APSED adoption and well into its first phase (2005–2010) (Coker et al. 2011). The effort by those within SEARO and the WPRO was to capture this financial and political enthusiasm to roll out national plans on pandemic influenza preparedness as a means by which to test and develop the five program areas under APSED. By directing national and regional resources to pandemic influenza preparedness, especially to the ongoing avian influenza outbreaks, event-based and early-warning surveillance and response could be tested in real time to provide insight on health system capacity in general. Furthermore, gaps in resources, diagnostics, and communication could be identified and directly support countries experiencing the ongoing AI outbreaks (Wilsmore et al. 2010).

At the same time as APSED's development, the UN Development Programme in New York had been funded to establish the Highly Pathogenic Avian Influenza Program, the function of which was to promote coordination of surveillance and detection processes in-country between animal health and human health. In the region there was a flurry of national pandemic preparedness plans, regional collaborative networks on virus sharing and diagnostics, and local training and communication about influenza outbreaks. The prevailing concern then and now was whether all this investment would flow into other priority diseases in the region—that is, whether best practices and networks would develop to inform and benefit the region in the more specific areas of IHR core capacity and wider areas of regional collaboration. Interestingly, at multiple training events between 2008 and 2010 led by ASEAN member states as part of the APT EID Programme, for example, on training of laboratory verification practices or fieldwork epidemiology training on infection control, the author heard the common advice provided to ministries of health that the influenza training and case study material should be adapted to suit the needs of addressing more local diseases such as Japanese encephalitis, TB, malaria, and dengue. The idea of adapting influenza preparedness for endemic cases and the crossover between addressing endemic diseases and preparing for the novel outbreaks was regularly voiced.

The 2010 APSED evaluation noted much of the above but did not provide a definitive finding on IHR readiness across the two regions at the point of review (Heywood and Moussavi 2010: 31). The APSED review noted that the evaluation of this indicator "was somewhat hampered by there not being a systematic database of capacity building support provided by the program" (43). At the same time, the review noted that the impediment to producing measurable outputs to judge the impact of APSED was in part to do with regional diversity, which could not be altered. The review suggested that what could and needed to be altered was the administrative differences between the two regional offices. Trust between the two offices, it was noted, was not yet in place to attach independent monitoring and evaluation to APSED programs (15). This is an important point I return to in chapter 6.

These concerns aside, the conclusion of the 2010 review was that the biregional strategy of regional engagement was a political strength in terms of a wide involvement of (state) stakeholders (Heywood and Moussavi 2010). The first-phase APSED document was deliberately framed to emphasize networks and collaboration over technical applications for measurement and comparison (WPRO 2005, 2010). Tailored to a regional context, the review found that IHR compliance was primarily conceptualized in the APSED first phase as strengthening national health systems: the connection to the region was that national capacity could be strong only if there was equally strong regional capacity. The achievement of global public health security was presented as depending, to a large degree, upon how successful regions develop and sustain "functional national and regional systems and capacities for managing emerging diseases and acute public health events and emergencies" (Li and Kasai 2011). As such, emphasis on the benefit of APSED went further than "just" building capacity in response to pandemics: "APSED outlines an approach to all emerging infectious diseases—from cholera, dengue and leptospirosis to the ever-present threat of pandemic influenza" (WPRO 2010: 12). Aligning APSED with regional health security was instrumental in persuading states to commit themselves to implementing the first phase (2005–2010). As such, the political cooperation facilitated through the first phase of APSED was vital (Heywood and Moussavi 2010: 9).

Conclusion

The first APSED phase established three regional dynamics critical to the implementation of the IHR. First, it moved beyond the structural separation of the WHO. APSED was a novel attempt to coordinate communication and engagement across two regions that were geographically linked by structural separation under the WHO management framework. This attempt, in and of itself, was a unique development for the WHO and for regional partnership concerning disease outbreak response and detection. It points to the extent to which the impact of SARS and H5N1, followed by the adoption of the revised IHR, led to a regional departure from politics as usual (at least temporarily). APSED was designed to offer something to all members—from those ready to meet IHR core capacities to those a long way behind. Inclusion of diseases endemic to the region to test the applicability of the IHR core capacities was one local adaption provided to entice coordination and relevance across the membership. However, this inclusion was mostly informal in practice. Given the variety of state capacity and health system strength, the contention that arose was whether APSED should be doing more than (just) assisting states with meeting IHR core capacities.

Second, APSED sought the inclusion of regional political institutions such as ASEAN and APT in order to promote additional structural and institutional opportunities for partnership and dialogue among its SEARO and WPRO states. Crucially, the ASEAN secretariat was invited to the meetings organized around the five APSED programs, which led to coordination between the APT EID Programme and the APSED phase by 2008 (APT Health Ministers Meeting 2008). This created, for ASEAN states in particular (as explored in the next chapter), an additional political and diplomatic commitment to APSED via ASEAN obligations. ASEAN states were no longer participating in APSED as individual WPRO or SEARO member states but also as ASEAN member states cognizant of their commitments to ASEAN. There was no doubt from all interviewed, whether located in SEARO, the WPRO, the ASEAN secretariat, or APSED TAG, that ASEAN's inclusion in APSED made a difference on national-level discussions of APSED among the ASEAN membership.

Third, APSED tailored its approach, working methods, and priorities to suit regional needs and sensitivities, with a premium placed on building regional interests while respecting key principles (such as noninterference). Cooperation was largely achieved by the avoidance of measurable targets on all 48-member states, but this left it vulnerable to critique. Those skeptical of the regional focus and who prefer a more global approach to IHR core capacity compliance pointed to precisely this lack of measurable targets in the first phase of APSED. Those skeptical of the securitization lens adopted in the region to promote health system strengthening to meet the IHR core capacities pointed to how APSED progressed a particular vision of IHR readiness that focused on detecting particular outbreaks, for example, avian influenza, rather than building detection systems that could improve overall detection and readiness. Those skeptical of the compliance pull of APSED in any form highlight the fact that in 2010 states still had live bird markets and there was little regional oversight into these markets' compliance with health protocols to limit the spread of disease. Collectively, these critiques point to a core tension: cooperation across the program areas required minimal political interference but maximum political support.

Measuring an individual state's commitment to the principles of alert, response, and verification being promoted under APSED is necessary, and it is the topic of the next chapter. However, before we go down the path of measurement, it is important to stand back and assess what APSED was set up to achieve in the first phase. As this chapter has demonstrated, the first thing to note is that it was not inevitable that APSED would be able to unite a broad selection of diverse member states across two large regions to understand and prepare for the core capacities required under the revised IHR. The revised IHR were four months old when APSED was approved. Inevitably, the first phase created dissatisfaction and genuine concern about the compliance pull of APSED. In response to these concerns during the first five years, we saw the layering of more institutional cohesion, not less. APSED did not disband, nor did it continue with minimal political engagement.

APSED's purpose was to tailor the revised IHR to regional circumstances. This created the possibility of coordinated behavioral change. It is to this point that I now turn—behavioral change in disease surveillance and response in Southeast Asia. In the next chapter I will show why the APSED initiative should be associated with positive changes in actual state behavior when it comes to reporting on infectious disease outbreaks.

CHAPTER FIVE

Surveillance and Reporting in Practice

As APSED was being developed and rolled out, ASEAN's Emerging Infectious Diseases Programme was entering its second phase (2007–2010) in partnership with the ASEAN Plus Three states, China, Japan, and South Korea. This program focused on three priorities that were closely aligned with APSED's and the IHR's core goals: establishing a shared event management website that would be used to normalize the dissemination of outbreak detection information, encouraging information sharing between states, and prioritizing communication around emerging infectious diseases. APSED and APT cooperation came together around three (of APSED's five) shared priorities: surveillance and detection, information sharing between members, and risk communication (APT Health Ministers Meeting 2008; WPRO 2005). As discussed in the previous chapter, this relationship established a common regional approach that crossed bureaucratic boundaries. Since ASEAN's members included states from both the SEARO and WPRO, its inclusion added another layer of local institutionalism that was practiced in finding consensus and diluted the potential SEARO-WPRO divide. ASEAN was able to fulfill this supportive role in part because of the constructive role played by its own secretariat. As previously mentioned, ASEAN health ministers had expressed their support for the health security agenda and the revised IHR, and as early as 2006 they had referred to APSED as an opportunity to expand and, crucially, attract funds to support these programs.

Taking this as a mandate, the ASEAN secretariat helped guide the ministerial focus to consider what was needed to achieve IHR compliance and to progress broader health cooperation goals. The secretariat satisfied the need to convey that changed practices and compliance with the IHR revisions were necessary and ought not to be prohibitively expensive. As one ASEAN official explained:

> Everyone [states] wants the best labs. States go around saying the revised IHR
> means they need BioSafety Level 4 labs. We bring them back from that demand

to help them see first what they really need is a structure to detect disease in the first place. Do their health clinics in a remote location know to contact their Ministry of Health if they see some symptoms that are different? Do their Ministry of Health officials in the urban areas know who to contact if they are being told about these odd symptoms in a remote location? What process do Ministry of Health officials have for confirmation? For finding out more information? Can a neighboring state get there faster to help with samples, verification? These are the conversations we are having right now. (Anonymous 2011c)

Within this context, the ASEAN secretariat helped facilitate interaction among member states, the WHO, and donors, giving rise to a better shared understanding of what was needed to address the problem of infectious disease outbreaks and how this might be achieved. In this, of course, the ASEAN secretariat was strongly supported by APSED.

Whatever the problems associated with APSED's first phase (see chap. 4), both the 2010 review and the general opinion of member states were positive about the effects the framework was having on regional cooperation. Shortfalls in individual state capacities across the five APSED program areas were repeatedly acknowledged, but there was also a shared view that this did not diminish the underlying commitment of states to progress toward compliance with the IHR core capacities. One particularly significant illustration of this increasing commitment was changes to reporting behavior with respect to disease outbreak events. In this chapter, I show *how* the behavior of Southeast Asian states changed with respect to outbreak reporting, and I explain why progress in this area was a significant indication of regional commitment to outbreak response.

This chapter proceeds in two parts. First, I present how I have located and coded outbreak reports in the region between 1996 and 2010. I have studied how ASEAN states have conducted their detection and reporting on both novel and endemic diseases (to the region) and traced trends in reporting patterns up to the end of the first phase of APSED (2010). In doing so, I differentiate between those outbreaks reported by the state (i.e., official ministry channels) and those reported by informal channels such as the media, NGOs, and internet disease surveillance platforms. This retrospective analysis traces the region's evolving engagement with surveillance performance and identifies change over time, from 1996 up to the review of APSED in 2010.

In the second part of the chapter, I discuss three trends in the reporting behavior of Southeast Asian states during this period. First, overall, ASEAN states improved their reporting performance, and this improved performance reached across both EIDs and diseases endemic to the region. Novel outbreak events including Nipah in 1998 and SARS in 2003, not to mention the increased prevalence of dengue outbreaks in the region since the mid-1990s, demonstrate how regional priorities had (already) been shifting in communicating disease outbreaks before the adoption of the revised IHR. Second, some disease outbreaks attracted higher levels of reporting than others, and the level of political interest appears to be determinative. There was a clear upward trend toward reporting disease outbreaks of local and international significance before 2005, but state-issued reports accelerated between 2005 and 2010. The introduction of the revised IHR followed by APSED, at the same time as the regional outbreak of H5N1 in humans, saw a swift uptake in states regularly reporting disease outbreak events. Notably, I find that even with the case of H5N1, where there was high media and international interest in suspected human infections, state-level reporting *consistently* outpaced informal reports. Third, the WHO's coverage of disease outbreak events in the region was skewed toward EID events and away from endemic outbreaks. The region's adoption of "health security" had already begun to change reporting behavior, and most ASEAN states were comfortable with adopting the revised IHR because they had themselves accepted the need to act in this way and viewed it as being in their interests.

Progress in the detection and open communication of outbreak events at the regional level is reflective, I suggest, of both the collective understanding of regional health security described earlier and individual state responsibility to contribute to regional health security. The adoption of the revised IHR was conceptualized as part of the regional undertaking to improving performance in this area and was referred to in both APSED and APT EID agendas. Enhanced cooperation in the area of surveillance was specifically emphasized in the first phase of APSED (2005–2010) and APT EID (2006–2009). The shift in reporting trends was certainly assisted, if not made possible, by the supportive networks established by APSED and the APT mechanism, which tailored global norms to regional interests and sensitivities and normalized participation.

Tracing outbreak reports in the region over fourteen years demonstrates a strong trend toward more open and prompt communication of disease outbreaks and enhanced freedom to report. However, as I stress in this chapter and chapter 6, although the overall trends are progressive, individual performance was mixed. Not all countries consistently report, some diseases are not detected or reported at their suspected infection rate, and states do not have uniform procedures for reporting suspected versus verified outbreak events.

There is, therefore, variation both among countries (some performing better than others) and within countries (some outbreaks reported more than others by the same state). Of course, variation like this is to be expected, given that the political context for each outbreak will be different and so too will be the epidemiological and technical context. Reporting performance, after all, is shaped by a combination of both political and technical factors. Cooperation in disease surveillance and detection requires technical and material capacity but also the political will to be transparent and allow free communication (S. Davies 2012). In examining the reporting behavior of ASEAN states over time, we can observe that the process and procedure for *verifying* outbreak events has evolved differently: states still appear to internalize their reporting responsibilities differently. It may be surmised that the trend toward enhanced detection and reporting remains at most risk in two areas: follow-up verification of initial disease outbreak reports and confronting the political situations that affect state capacity to detect and respond.

Tracing Surveillance and Response

To understand the changing performance of ASEAN member states in disease surveillance and response, I traced surveillance reports relating to the ASEAN states (seven WPRO and three SEARO members) from 1996 to 2010.[1] I examined reports for a broad range of infectious diseases: human infections from avian influenza (including H5N1 and H7N9), cholera, dengue (including dengue hemorrhagic fever), Japanese encephalitis, Nipah, "other" (see definition on p. 119), respiratory infections, SARS, and IHR 1 and IHR 2 category outbreaks (defined under the IHR 2005 Annex 2 list). Two sites were sourced for reports of disease outbreak events. The first was the WHO's *Disease Outbreak News* website (this site began regular reporting from 1996, and many of the disease reports were not limited to IHR [1969] listed diseases). I supplemented these reports with the WHO *Weekly Epidemiological Report* of outbreak events in the region—this source was available for use in the early years prior to all reports shifting to *DON*. By 2000, *DON* was overtaking *WER* reports in terms of real-time alerts. The second site I used for reports of infectious disease outbreak events was the ProMED-mail server (Program for Monitoring Emerging Diseases, or PMM), an infectious disease surveillance platform. I will briefly detail the rationale for selecting the PMM as the alternative outbreak-reporting source to the WHO before discussing how I selected the countries and diseases examined here.

One of the most reliable open sources for immediate reports of outbreak events from a variety of primary sources, which include local media, public health ministries, and individual informants, is the global disease surveillance reporting system ProMED (Grein et al. 2000; Madoff and Woodall 2005; Castillo-Salgedo 2010). During the 1990s, internet technology inspired the creation of global surveillance networks. Web-based health surveillance tools, such as the text mining of media reports for disease outbreak events (e.g., the EU Joint Research Centre MedISys, Google's Health Map), led to the creation of disease alert lists that are distributed to subscribers to receive and report outbreak events (e.g., PMM, GPHIN, and HealthMap). ProMED was created by the Federation of American Scientists in 1994, and then teamed up with the International Society of Infectious Diseases in 1999 to expand its coverage and capacity. ProMED was among the first internet disease surveillance networks to develop regional contacts and experts in multiple languages and regions to access local reports on disease events. These networks provided a portal for receiving information about outbreak events from media, individual scientists, health practitioners, and ministries of health. The listserv is moderated by experts to ensure accuracy and disseminate to a wide readership across universities, health ministries, hospitals, laboratories, and international organizations, including the WHO. This moderation means that every report received from a "source" or detected by text mining software is analyzed for authenticity. As a result, the PMM is known for its accuracy, with its initial reports of suspected outbreaks often being verified by the state in follow-up reports (Madoff and Woodall 2005; Collier 2010). Initially, the PMM did not have the text-mining algorithm strength or staff of the Public Health Agency of Canada's GPHIN or European Union's MedISys.[2] However, the PMM's principal contribution has always been its expertise in moderating reports before dissemination—this means that no report is issued on the server until an expert has assessed it and judged it to be relevant and factual (Madoff and Woodall 2005: 725–727).

The PMM also has a reputation for political independence—subscribers are provided nonpartisan information and analysis of outbreak events that may otherwise be overlooked were it not for the PMM's network of "insider informants" using the system to communicate outbreak events (Madoff and Woodall 2005; Brownstein et al. 2008). It is because of this reputation for being an early informant on outbreak events, coupled with its archive function that dates back to its first year of introduction (1994) and publication of outbreaks in English (which have been translated from their original language) that I selected it as the comparative source to the WHO's *DON*: it allows me to compare official and unofficial reporting from sources separate to the state.

Alternative reporting sources not selected include the Global Public Health Information Network, another early first in real-time surveillance networks (created in 1996) and developed by the Public Health Agency of Canada in cooperation with WHO headquarters. The GPHIN remains a primary informant for the WHO of outbreak events (events that may not have [yet] been reported directly to the WHO by the affected state) (Anonymous 2010n, 2014). Similar in method to the PMM, the GPHIN has human analysts with language proficiency in Arabic, Farsi, English, Spanish, Russian, Chinese, Portuguese, and French who sift through thousands of reports produced daily to determine which require being placed on the subscriber-only alert page (which can also be emailed to subscribers). From 1996 to 2005, its reports were primarily issued to subscribers and are therefore not more widely accessible. This ruled out GPHIN as the primary source for this study. Health-Map is a free access internet surveillance network that analyzes media reports on a scale similar to GPHIN and also reports from other surveillance internet providers such as MedISys (an EU Joint Research Centre project), ProMED, the WHO, and Google Trends for keyword search, including blogs and social media sites, to produce real-time alerts of disease outbreak with color codes indicating source reliability (which entails "last minute" human moderation prior to posting) (Brownstein et al. 2008). HealthMap and MedISys have comprehensive archive search functions, but these began only in 2008, making them less than suitable.

Within the Asia Pacific region, the PMM has a record of "first reports." It was the first to communicate the Nipah virus outbreak in Malaysia in 1999 after an informal source provided the server with laboratory findings (Madoff and Woodall 2005); the server was one of the first to report that the atypical pneumonia cases in China in 2003 were in fact a new virus; PMM moderators provided trace reports of H5N1 outbreaks in the region, including during the period when the Indonesian government threatened to stop reporting suspected events to the WHO; and, farther to the west, the PMM reported the first Middle East Respiratory Syndrome (MERS) case in Middle East in 2012 (again, before the WHO) (S. Davies 2017). The PMM reporting partners in the region include the Mekong Basin Disease Surveillance Network, whose secretariat has sought a close reporting relationship with the PMM (Maddoff and Woodall 2005; Anonymous 2012c). Finally, in terms of event reporting accuracy, the PMM has been measured at 91% (Freifeld et al. 2008: 150).

The PMM relies on individual informers to provide it with information about outbreak events that may not be immediately published on sites like the WHO's

Disease Outbreak News website (the WHO must wait for state permission to go public). Therefore, the PMM, given its emergence close to the same time as the WHO's *DON*, coupled with its reputation for publishing reports not always officially communicated, provides insight into which outbreak events are readily communicated to the WHO by official channels and which take a little more time to reach the WHO—if they do at all. The PMM reports thus provide the most informative contrast to WHO *DON* reports for two reasons. First, because it is necessary to compare the outbreak reports being received formally by the WHO from states with the suspected reports more likely to be issued by the PMM on that same country. An increase in reporting to the WHO may still not indicate the true extent of suspected outbreak events occurring in a country. The PMM provides an additional measure to test states' own behavioral change in detecting and reporting outbreak events. Second, because comparison of reporting sources provides the chance to analyze which outbreaks are communicated and shared with the WHO, which are verified by the state but not reported to the WHO, and which are not reported or verified by officials.

The rationale for disease selection was driven by the need to study the reporting history for a combination of (revised) IHR Annex 2 diseases. The revised IHR have three columns under Annex 2 that list the types of disease that the instrument may cover and therefore require states to detect and report outbreak events. The first column of the revised IHR Annex 2 refers to diseases that are "unusual and unexpected" that require immediate notification (also known as IHR Category 1): smallpox, polio, human influenza (any type), and SARS. Because I was tracing these reports from 1996 and some of these were not included under the IHR prior to its revision, I wanted to capture reports of these diseases individually. Therefore, for reports on influenza, for example, I introduced two reporting categories to capture all the reports: avian infections in humans (which dated back to 1997 in the region) and respiratory influenza (which included all other seasonal reports, including H1N1). H1N1 only shifted to entry as an IHR 1 category report *after* its formal declaration as a Public Health Emergency of International Concern. The second column in IHR Annex 2 refers to any event of international concern that is not listed in the left or right column in Annex 2 (IHR Category 2). I collected any report that referred to an incident that may have been an IHR Category 2 event or a PHEIC that was not otherwise defined. However, these entries were placed under IHR Category 2 only from 2007. Until 2007, Category 2 events were included in the "other" category—which tabled any suspected outbreak report that had not yet been identified and verified by the state (or a laboratory) to the PMM or WHO.

Crucially, the revised IHR replaced the earlier categorization of specific diseases to be reported with broader disease categories that may pose a risk to international public health and demanded that states be cognizant of the definition "public health emergency of international concern" in deciding whether to report. Under the revised IHR the "mere presence of cases of these diseases does not automatically require notification or automatically fulfil any of the four criteria," but, notably, regions were allowed to expand this list if they wished.[3] Therefore, I kept track of reports of outbreak events identified as significant by the region—which led to inclusion of Nipah and SARS (it is not listed under IHR Category 1, as it was detected in 2003—before the adoption of revised IHR) as discreet disease categories. And I did not focus on just the IHR (1969) and (2005) categories but reports for two diseases endemic in both SEARO and the WPRO—neither of which necessitate regular reporting to the WHO but are considered important diseases that fall under the regional health security definition in APSED literature—dengue (including dengue hemorrhagic fever) and Japanese encephalitis.

To properly understand patterns of disease reporting in the region, we need to include diseases considered important by the region even if they do not make it onto the global radar. That is because we need to understand whether the IHR skewed reporting toward those diseases that matter most globally and away from regional priorities. At the same time, IHR-notifiable diseases are, thankfully, rare. To comprehend how a program like APSED was making a difference, we need to understand how states understood their IHR reporting obligations versus the day-to-day function of reducing infectious disease burden against endemic diseases. Tracing states' public communication of a wide category of diseases—novel and endemic—provides insight into whether states are enhancing their performance only for the events likely to attract international interest or whether they are able to cross the divide and build capacity to address both emerging and endemic infectious diseases. Finally, tracing reporting performance from 1996 to 2010, for a wide category of diseases, allows us to understand the degree to which events such as SARS and H5N1, diplomatic events such as adoption of the IHR and creation of APSED, and donor funding served as important triggers for changing state performance.

To evaluate the performance of every state over this period, the ideal data entry process is to trace the time between initial report of outbreak and laboratory confirmation of the same outbreak. Similar studies have been conducted (e.g., Chan et al. 2010; Kluberg et al. 2016), and I relied upon some of their insights in defining my outbreak categories. However, in my research, I found that few countries (with exception of Singapore) consistently provided open-source data back to 1996. Whether due to problems of scale or capacity, many of the countries examined here compiled outbreak events and simply reported total (confirmed) cases on a monthly basis through their Ministry of Health websites (and many did not provide this information online and in English until early to mid-2000s). Therefore, I found it very difficult to trace individual outbreak reports from suspected to verified in most instances. Details provided on location, identity of infected individual(s), and suspected illnesses were not often an identical match to confirmed reports later released by the state or WHO. Therefore, I could not trace the time (days/months) between outbreak and verification, which is a limit of this study and a point I return to in the next chapter.

The few instances of crossover reporting, where cholera reports were orig-inally reported as "diarrhoea" or "other" and Nipah outbreaks were reported initially as Japanese encephalitis or "other," were corrected when triangulation was possible. With the exception of the H5N1 human infections, disease out-breaks in animals are not included in this study because of project constraints and relevance for the project—therefore the Ebola Reston virus outbreak in the Philippines in 2008 (arguably, a significant event of public health concern) is recorded under IHR Category 1. Likewise, I did not refer to the WHO's Global Influenza Surveillance Network (GISN) for respiratory influenza reports, mainly because the GISN does provide data for all the ASEAN countries back to 1996. In this framework, data collection begins earlier and traces the relationship between informal and official reporting for "unusual or unexpected out-breaks."

Endemic diseases in the region such as dengue and Japanese encephalitis were chosen over, for example, chikungunya, malaria, TB, or hand, foot, and mouth, because these reflect the priorities for improved surveillance identified by the region itself (WPRO 2005; ASEAN 2007). In addition, I considered the question of what constituted sudden and unexpected outbreaks, in accordance with the definition of PHEIC under the revised IHR. Dengue and dengue hem-orrhagic fever had been repeatedly singled out by both the WPRO and SEARO as a disease steadily spreading across the Asia Pacific, including cities and the urban sprawl, dramatically increasing the caseloads and fatality rates (WPRO 2005). Furthermore, both regional offices have argued that containment and response require active surveillance to curb their spread. Dengue hemorrhagic fever is the leading cause of hospitalization and death among children in the East Asian region (WHO 2017d). Indeed, after the IHR revisions in 2005, dengue hemorrhagic fever was identified by the WPRO as being a possible IHR Category 1 disease (WPRO 2005). The rise in dengue fever during this period also made it an important inclusion for identifying how the region was reporting and responding to a regional endemic disease (as a contrast to unexpected disease outbreak events).

Japanese encephalitis was chosen for the same reason: because it has periods of endemic outbreak (Coker et al. 2011).[4] In addition, it has a complex relationship with Nipah virus in that Japanese encephalitis is often attributed as cause for infection when it may in fact be Nipah virus, which is listed by SEARO as an infectious disease of utmost importance for testing surveillance and response (SEARO 2011). Nipah is a henipavirus that can be transmitted from pigs to humans (as in Malaysia, where the disease was first discovered in 1998) or from fruit bats to humans, with reports of limited human-to-human transfer in cases in Bangladesh and India since 2001. It is deemed to be a disease of public health concern largely because it infects a wide range of animals, which transmit to humans, possibly from human to human, and infections are linked to high mortality with no known vaccine or cure (WHO 2017e). Therefore, the capacity to detect Japanese encephalitis is widely considered by some within the region to be a vital surveillance capacity (Anonymous 2010a). This disease is also very difficult to diagnose outside of the laboratory, causing time lags in its identification that could enable its spread.

Entries for disease outbreaks were tabulated in the relevant year and the relevant country reported as the location of the outbreak, and the report would then be tabled as a WHO-sourced report; an official report—one sourced from the PMM but the outbreak report originated from a Ministry of Health official or news release; and an informal report—one provided by an individual or a news report with no confirmation or response from official government channels. This distinction is of primary importance for analyzing reports, especially from the PMM. The argument in the literature on internet surveillance platforms like the PMM is that states are increasingly "second in line" to report disease outbreaks, that often the first news comes from media sources that have detected a disease outbreak rumor. It is when media agencies get hold of these reports that states will then either confirm or deny the report, by releasing details of an outbreak investigation or providing lab diagnostic results (Grein et al. 2000; Madoff and Woodall 2005; Brownstein et al. 2008). Understanding how often states are playing "catch-up" to rumors is crucial to identifying what steps they are taking to improve their surveillance and response in order to, in turn, improve their risk communication: reassuring the community of timely response and containment, as well as reassuring neighboring countries and the international community that the state is cognizant of the outbreak (Rodier 2007).

Tracing the number of outbreaks first reported by informal rather than official government sources, and whether there are changes over time, tells us how states understand their role in surveillance and response. Any report concerning a possible disease outbreak event in the relevant countries selected, reported by government, new media or "other" (e.g., email communication) was recorded. Finally, I tracked disease events that received all three reports—first informal, then official, and then WHO—as well as those disease events that received only one (informal, official, or WHO) against those that received only two (informal and official, official and WHO, informal and WHO). The purpose of this multiple disease reporting category was to trace the most "popular" form of disease reporting, to track states' progress against other disease "notifiers," and to understand how these reporting types may differ across the diseases I tracked.

A final point on the method is how a "new" report was identified and entered during outbreaks, particularly in the case of cholera, dengue, H5N1 in humans, SARS, and respiratory influenza. Generally, the approach was to impose a geographical and time limit before identifying an outbreak as new. Time lags for disease outbreaks generally followed a 14-day rule (Chan et al. 2010). If there was a 14-day lag in reporting a disease outbreak (i.e., no new reports or reports of disease spread), the next outbreak of same disease would be classified as new. The goal here was not always to trace the progression of an actual case but to trace the progression of state reporting compared to the progression of informal reporting behavior. For example, if a cholera outbreak had spread but was still identified as being linked by strain and geography to the original source and reported within 14 days of first report, then there was no new entry. The same approach was adopted for dengue, with geographic spread (beyond two provinces/states) and time lapse (i.e., more than two weeks) being the primary guide for discerning whether a new report was warranted. If, however, there were a number of dengue hemorrhagic fever cases emerging from a dengue outbreak, this was entered as a new event because of higher mortality associated with the fever cases. The same fortnightly approach was taken to reporting H5N1 human infections and influenza, as with dengue and cholera, with one exception if a report identified the outbreak was in a new area or geographically distant from previous areas reported.

Regional Surveillance Reporting Trends

The data yielded three core findings. First, overall ASEAN states improved their reporting performance, and that improved performance reached across both EIDs and diseases endemic to the region. Official reporting behavior, in particular, over the past 14 years showed marked improvement for reporting endemic and epidemic outbreaks. Second, some disease outbreaks attracted higher levels of reporting than others, and the level of political interest appears to be determinative. Even the more recalcitrant reporting state will report at some point an outbreak that attracts regional concern at the political level while it will tend to be laxer about reporting endemic diseases that do not attract such levels of interest. Third, the WHO's coverage of disease outbreak events in the region is skewed toward EID events and away from endemic outbreaks. This is not surprising, but it does highlight the importance of regional-level projects that are dedicated to capacity building for those diseases that create high health burdens in the region, lest a critical gap emerge between the global priorities pursued by the WHO and the challenges that confront particular regions. Such gaps could, of course, contribute to noncompliance with the IHR. If reporting to the WHO under the revised IHR is the end goal, the path toward this is ensuring that global expectations align more closely with regional realities.

Overall, then, regional-level programming that encourages reporting of the regular endemic events, such as dengue, appears to normalize detection and reporting and extends these behaviors to the events that are of international concern like H5N1. Other studies of the WPRO and SEARO have detected similar encouraging results in how surveillance and response, one of the eight core capacities of the revised IHR, has dramatically progressed in a short time (Chan et al. 2010; Kluberg et al. 2016). This study complements these findings but extends them in arguing that the key to understanding them lies in the cooperation between APSED and APT EID programming, which encouraged regional selection of core capacities under the revised IHR that were of political importance to the region. The combination of the global drive toward meeting IHR core capacities and the critical regional-led efforts to tailor such processes to regional priorities and sensitivities explains why the progress was so impressive in such a short time (if variable across cases). I will turn now to each of these findings.

Regional Reporting

Recent studies have demonstrated an overall improvement in the timeliness of confirmation (Chan et al. 2010; Kluberg et al. 2016) and specific disease reporting in relation to influenza (Coker et al. 2011). In studying the surveillance and reporting core capacities for the five WHO regions since the revised IHR, Chan et al. (2010) found that the time between outbreak detection and verification had been significantly reduced in the WPRO and Eastern Mediterranean Regional Office (EMRO) regions, with SEARO also demonstrating some improvement. Chan and colleagues surmised that the spread of avian influenza (2004–2008 were the most intense years) at the time may have propelled these regions' readiness and engagement with the revised IHR (Chan et al. 2010). A few years later, Sheryl Kluberg and colleagues replicated Chan et al.'s study. Kluberg and colleagues found that the WPRO region had continued to improve its disease surveillance and response capacity; SEARO and EMRO had also made improvements but not at the pace they had made up to 2010. The study concluded that, "despite regional disparities in timeliness of disease discovery, all regions showed some improvement. Variability between regions probably resulted from a combination of differences in culture, Internet availability, and previous outbreak experiences" (Kluberg et al. 2016).

Official (O)—state-based—reporting since 1996 has experienced the most significant growth as the primary source of outbreak event reporting among the ASEAN states. States are now the primary sources of outbreak events—providing the reports before informal (I) reports: before the media report suspect events, before individual communications to internet surveillance networks like PMM, and before (in recent years) social media. The overall regional trend has seen an improvement in the *official* reporting of all disease outbreaks, while there has been an increase in informal reports—but the rise in this source is modest compared to the growth in the state sector (figure 5.1).

There are two important points to note about these data. First, official reporting in the region has dramatically increased—at least fourfold—in 10 years (from 40 reports in 2000 to 180 in 2010). Second, informal reports have *not* experienced the same upward trajectory. The reduction in non-state-issued informal reports is, interestingly, consistent with a prediction that was made by surveillance and response advocates in the early years of promoting the

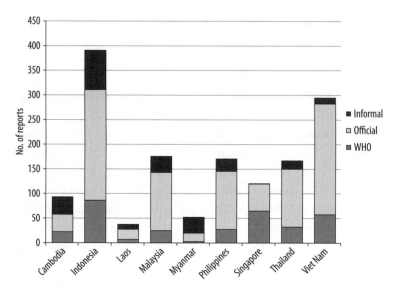

Figure 5.1. Total Source of Outbreak Reports in ASEAN, 1996–2010

revised IHR: if states managed to improve their information flow of disease outbreak events and report, there would be less need for informal reports, which would decline in prevalence. This was a message also conveyed in the APSED program and one that the author personally witnessed in the early years of program delivery within the region.

In Southeast Asia, the tendency has been for internet surveillance platforms to mostly report official notices on disease outbreaks (e.g., the PMM). States themselves are therefore the primary source because they are increasingly being proactive in their reporting. An alternative interpretation of the data is that reports by informal sources are subjected to greater state control via censorship and the punishment of those who issue unofficial reports—and that this explains their lack of growth. This has been evident in some situations, such as the Ebola outbreak in Guinea and MERS reports in Saudi Arabia. The possibility of growing state regulatory control on informal reports should not be disregarded in the ASEAN region, especially in those countries where the regime's control of the media could be described as intrusive (i.e., Cambodia, Laos, Myanmar, and Viet Nam). However, to date, among ASEAN states there is no evidence of such controls or of penalties being imposed on those who have informally reported an outbreak without state permission. By contrast, in the MERS and Ebola cases, there were immediate reports of states in the

Middle East and West Africa respectively engaging in precisely this sort behavior at the time of the public health emergency (S. Davies 2017). In short, were states acting against the sources of informal reports, we would have evidence of it.

In at least two countries, however, it has become common practice for unofficial news reporting of outbreaks to be sourced from official sources (Anonymous 2010b, 2010g). In both Cambodia and Viet Nam, officials tend to personally communicate information to the media to ensure that reports of outbreak events have a public official quoted within the report, giving the government some degree of control over messaging. In these cases, health ministries requested that they be sourced in any media report so that they can communicate the message that the government is aware of the outbreak and reassure the public that it is taking action. This indicates a high level of coordinated messaging between government and media; what is not clear in such a close relationship is how the media could respond to critical allegations outside the government regarding outbreak verification, response, and handling. However, if we compare these two states' rates of informal reports with those of the region's more democratic states such as the Philippines and Thailand (at the time), there is a striking similarity in the number and pattern of informal reports with formal reports (figures 5.2 and 5.3).

Myanmar, for most of the time during this study, was the most politically oppressive state when it came to media and internet freedoms (partial reforms in 2010 began to relax these restrictions very incrementally). The diseases in this country that were regularly reported informally were cholera and dengue, and there was one unconfirmed report of plague (figure 5.3). The diseases formally reported by Myanmar officials during the period between 2005 and 2010 were suspected H5N1, respiratory infection at the time of H1N1, polio, and dengue (figure 5.2). By no coincidence perhaps, each of these diseases is of priority to ASEAN (dengue), APSED (H5N1), and the IHR Emergency Committee (H1N1, polio), and reports may have been issued to demonstrate some compliance with the regional call for regular reporting.

Overall, the high volume of outbreak reports, whether from the WHO (see figure 5.4), the state, or an informal source, all point to the diseases of international concern receiving the most attention. This, however, indicates concern that global health security and viral sovereignty agendas were driving states to create surveillance and response procedures to satisfy global demands at the expense of health systems designed to meet specific national challenges or priorities. For example, while developing capacity in relation to EIDs, the same

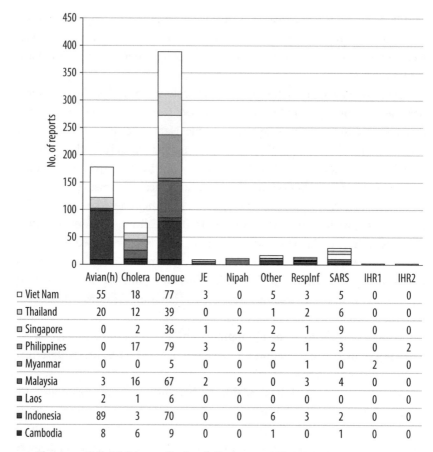

	Avian(h)	Cholera	Dengue	JE	Nipah	Other	RespInf	SARS	IHR1	IHR2
□ Viet Nam	55	18	77	3	0	5	3	5	0	0
□ Thailand	20	12	39	0	0	1	2	6	0	0
□ Singapore	0	2	36	1	2	2	1	9	0	0
▣ Philippines	0	17	79	3	0	2	1	3	0	2
▣ Myanmar	0	0	5	0	0	0	1	0	2	0
▪ Malaysia	3	16	67	2	9	0	3	4	0	0
▪ Laos	2	1	6	0	0	0	0	0	0	0
▪ Indonesia	89	3	70	0	0	6	3	2	0	0
▪ Cambodia	8	6	9	0	0	1	0	1	0	0

Figure 5.2. Official Disease Outbreak Reports in ASEAN Region, 1996–2010

state could not effectively detect and manage hand, foot, and mouth outbreaks (Calain 2007). Indeed, this was the primary concern of critics of APSED and the revised IHR in the region during this phase (Aldis 2008)—that although states were improving compliance with global norms, this was skewing their health policies away from local priorities. This is a point I return to on p. 133.

What Is Being Reported

As noted above, overall performance in official reporting behavior has become progressively stronger in Southeast Asia, but there is variation in performance from disease to disease. Official reports are substantially ahead of informal reports for AI human infection cases, dengue outbreaks, and respiratory infections, as well as during the SARS outbreak in 2003. For the four years examined,

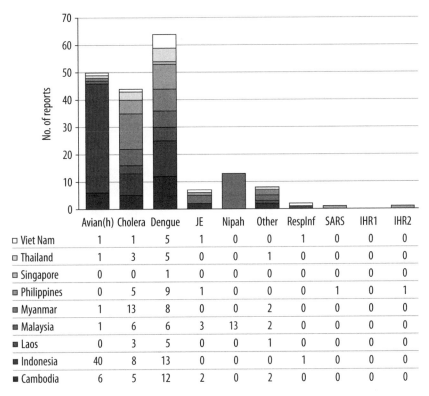

	Avian(h)	Cholera	Dengue	JE	Nipah	Other	RespInf	SARS	IHR1	IHR2
☐ Viet Nam	1	1	5	1	0	0	1	0	0	0
☐ Thailand	1	3	5	0	0	1	0	0	0	0
☐ Singapore	0	0	1	0	0	0	0	0	0	0
☐ Philippines	0	5	9	1	0	0	0	1	0	1
☐ Myanmar	1	13	8	0	0	2	0	0	0	0
☐ Malaysia	1	6	6	3	13	2	0	0	0	0
☐ Laos	0	3	5	0	0	1	0	0	0	0
☐ Indonesia	40	8	13	0	0	0	1	0	0	0
☐ Cambodia	6	5	12	2	0	2	0	0	0	0

Figure 5.3. Informal Disease Outbreaks Reported in ASEAN region, 1996–2010

IHR Category 1 and IHR Category 2 reveal strong state performance in reporting suspected outbreaks, in fact, well above the informal reports issued under the two categories. Though to a lesser extent, state reporting for cholera outbreaks was still strong (with the exception of Myanmar), though, notably, states no longer need to report cholera outbreaks under the revised IHR unless the outbreak is unusual and the country's IHR focal point suspects high risk of international transmission. The diseases with less impressive growth in detection and reporting (particularly compared to suspected numbers of infection) and less impressive official reporting compared to informal reports were Japanese encephalitis, Nipah, and "other" (figures 5.2, 5.3, and 5.4).

Dengue, followed by reports of avian influenza infection in humans, exhibited the greatest positive reporting trend with official reports outpacing informal reports (see figures 5.2 and 5.3). In fact, dengue reports exceeded all the other disease reports examined in this framework. Dengue also had the highest outbreak report record of all the diseases examined, which partly accounts for

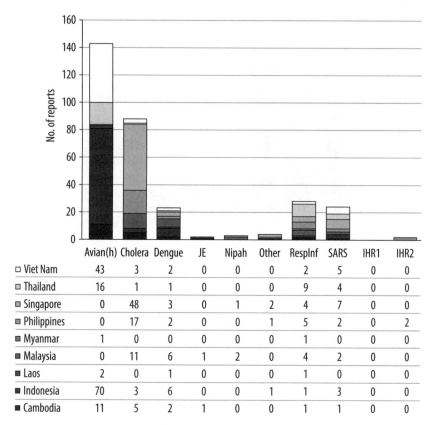

	Avian(h)	Cholera	Dengue	JE	Nipah	Other	RespInf	SARS	IHR1	IHR2
▢ Viet Nam	43	3	2	0	0	0	2	5	0	0
▢ Thailand	16	1	1	0	0	0	9	4	0	0
▢ Singapore	0	48	3	0	1	2	4	7	0	0
▣ Philippines	0	17	2	0	0	1	5	2	0	2
▪ Myanmar	1	0	0	0	0	0	1	0	0	0
▪ Malaysia	0	11	6	1	2	0	4	2	0	0
▪ Laos	2	0	1	0	0	0	1	0	0	0
▪ Indonesia	70	3	6	0	0	1	1	3	0	0
▪ Cambodia	11	5	2	1	0	0	1	1	0	0

Figure 5.4. WHO Reported Disease Outbreaks in ASEAN region, 1996–2010

the strong improvement in the official regional reporting trend. Dengue reports—and the coordination required to conduct dengue reports—is one of the "good news" stories of this framework. Given its regularity in the region, it also serves to (somewhat) counter the suggestion that a surveillance and reporting focus crowds out addressing regional endemic diseases over the "trendier" novel diseases like H5N1. Dengue has a long history in the Asian region; its incidence, and that of the deadly hemorrhagic fever, has made this disease the leading cause of hospitalization and death among children and adults in the region (WHO 2017f).

Dengue surveillance was starting to gather pace at the start of this study in 1996. In 1995, the WHO's director-general expressed concern about the increasing dengue outbreaks in the Asian region in a report to the Executive Board on the importance of developing event-based surveillance (as opposed to indicator-based surveillance) to detect and contain outbreaks (WHA EB95/61 1995: 1–2). The 1998 outbreak in the region, on record as one of the worst outbreaks for cases and deaths (WHO *WER* 73[36] 1998: 273), saw 21 official reports, 190 WHO reports, and 9 informal reports, with 7 of those informal reports never verified. Then, in 2001, the official report tally was 17, no reports were issued by the WHO, and there were 2 informal reports. The WHO reported at the time that it believed that many outbreaks were not being reported (WHO *WER* 77[6] 2001), and, in the same year, the WHO created DengueNet, an event-based surveillance network for reporting dengue outbreaks. The principle behind DengueNet was that "case reports should be transmitted from the local level to the state/provincial and then national level, and from there to WHO for international reporting and use. However, [at present] the reporting of dengue/DHF is not standardized. Epidemiological and laboratory data are often collected by different institutions and reported in different formats, resulting in delay and comparability problems at regional and international levels" (WHO *WER* 77[36]).

DengueNet was established in 2003 to gather reports from the WPRO and SEARO (Indonesia, Thailand, and Viet Nam agreed to assist the WHO in the 2003 DengueNet meeting in region); with WHO Collaborating Labs to assist in diagnosis and WHO headquarters assuming responsibility for administering the network. Two events overtook WHO management of this network—SARS and then H5N1. Interestingly, ASEAN still promoted dengue awareness among its membership, and dengue was listed in the first APSED documents—from 2005—as part of health security preparedness. As figure 5.2 shows, despite WHO's concerns in 2001 that states were not reporting the volume of dengue outbreaks, reports from ministries of health since 2000 had steadily increased among ASEAN membership (see figure 5.2). The WHO, however, did not issue reports on dengue via *DON* during this period (see figure 5.4). Informal reports (not confirmed by ministry, see figure 5.3) of dengue also increased during this period—though not at the same rate as official reporting (with the exception of Cambodia and Myanmar—where informal reports outnumbered their official reports from 1996 to 2010). Given that informal reports were so low for the majority of countries, it seems likely that health departments were in most instances leading the dengue surveillance and risk communication strategy.

The regularity of dengue reporting during this period should focus discussion on how to translate the gains in surveillance and reporting achieved for this disease to other endemic mosquito-borne diseases, such as malaria and Japanese encephalitis (pp. 133–134), without the time-consuming and costly process of laboratory diagnosis. One concern, however, is that, despite a massive increase in official reports, all mosquito-borne diseases remain difficult to diagnose and report at the suspected rate that they are *occurring*. This has led to further public relations exercises and public diplomacy initiatives such as the ASEAN Dengue Day (held every year on 15 June since 2010) and the Asia Pacific Leaders Malaria Alliance (created in 2013).

Within this generally positive picture, two countries stand out as bucking the trend: Cambodia and Myanmar. A third, Laos, stands out because of the very low level of reports overall. In all three cases, relatively weak performance reflected capacity difficulties for countries with high disease burdens and limited health systems. All three countries have governments with authoritarian tendencies, so it should also not be discounted that there is, possibly, political reluctance to officially communicate disease outbreaks to the population.

In the case of *avian influenza infection in humans*, the only inconsistency in the upward reporting trajectory was 2009, when informal reporting nearly reached the same level as official and WHO-confirmed reports (see figures 5.2, 5.3, and 5.4). Peak reporting for the region was in 2005 (see figure 5.2) and was mostly issued by official reports, with the WHO closely following.

The two most affected states, Indonesia and Viet Nam, had different reporting peaks. Official reports for Indonesia were at their highest in 2006 and 2007, while for Viet Nam it was 2004 and 2005. During this period there was always residual concern that Indonesia and Viet Nam were not promptly reporting outbreaks (ProMED report 20060824.2389). Viet Nam did have a dramatic lull in reporting in 2006—just 1 official report compared to 21 in the preceding year and 7 in the following year. Viet Nam's sudden drop during this period has been attributed to the political backlash within the country to the chicken cull that followed outbreak reports.

Indonesia's reporting lull for H5N1 actually came later than 2006. From 2008 to 2009 there was a sudden drop in the figures from 13 to 5 official reports and then an increase to 12 official reports in 2010. In 2009, this is the first and only time we see unofficial reports (10) outpace official reports (5) in Indonesia concerning H5N1. Given that it was in 2008 when the Indonesian minister of health announced a periodic ban on H5N1 case reporting to the WHO, this may explain the sudden media and ISRP interest in unverified reports of H5N1 "rumors" in 2009, coupled with the government's apparent reluctance to report cases. As noted above, officials in Jakarta—both WHO and Ministry of Health officials—observed that communication channels remained open during 2008 and 2009. During that time human infectious cases of H5N1 were reported in high numbers and came second only to dengue for the region in terms of regular reports of caseload. The fact is that, despite the dispute over virus sharing, reporting continued.

Of course, unlike dengue, the H5N1 human infections were not endemic, nor did they develop into a human-to-human infectious disease as had been feared. Indeed, others noted the volume of H5N1 reports emanating from within the region at the time (Shiffman 2006: 418; Coker et al. 2011: 607), and their concern was that the focus on surveillance, prevention, and treatment of avian influenza distracted expenditure and resources from detecting and treating diseases affecting the region in high numbers at the time, such as Japanese encephalitis, dengue, and even less publicized diseases such as malaria, rabies, tuberculosis, and chikungunya virus. An additional concern was whether the focus on H5N1 detection was actually assisting with detection in the fullest sense. One concern that came to the fore during the height of H5N1 was that the time-consuming task of testing whether individuals were infected with the H5N1 strain or "just" a common influenza strain took precious health system resources away from other problems.

Unsurprisingly, the only time we consistently see the WHO marginally ahead of official and informal reporting is with the reports of respiratory infections—those cases that received the greatest political attention at the highest levels. This pattern is largely attributable to the Global Infectious Disease Surveillance Network, now called the Global Influenza Surveillance and Response System (GISRS), that has been managed by the WHO since 1952. This system has been vital for coordinating national response and information on the transmission and mutation of virus strains. The GISN (now GISRS) collaborated with national laboratories and vaccine development in both developed and developing countries, particularly in the Asian region (Smith 2012). Indeed, one of the concerns about Indonesia's actions in 2007 was that withholding an H5N1 sample could have been the start of unravelling the GISN, which has always relied upon countries sharing influenza strains among 140-odd institutions—National Influenza Centres, six WHO Collaborating Labs, and four WHO Essential Regulatory Laboratories. The lack of country-level official reports on seasonal outbreaks was curious in that their annual pattern would be high enough to warrant some communication on patterns and type, but it appears that the region left reports for this particular infectious disease to the WHO *DON* (with exception of 2009, when official reports were at their highest level and all in reference to the H1N1 outbreak). It is also possible that these reports do not make it to the PMM unless the spike is unusual. This appears to be corroborated by the fact that informal reports were also rare and tended to focus only on "unusual" spikes in seasonal or novel respiratory infections, for example, among particular age groups, provinces, or locales that were perceived by local populations to be high caseload (which led to the report). Interestingly, these unofficial reports were nearly always followed up by an official report, with the exception of one suspected outbreak event in Indonesia.

By the time SARS broke out in 2003, ASEAN states had experienced successive years of dengue as well as the Nipah outbreak in 1999. SARS reinforced the learning earlier established—that effective risk communication required they speak with one voice during emergencies. Then during the H5N1 outbreak official reports—with the exception of one year in Indonesia—managed to outpace the rumor mill of informal reports. Moreover, confirmation of outbreak events was well paced, with the WHO regularly reporting verified outbreaks in follow-up to suspected outbreaks (see figure 5.4). However, this pace starts to diminish once we move beyond those diseases that captured international attention (e.g., SARS and H5N1) and those that have the diplomatic attention of the region (e.g., dengue). One of the main concerns among those watching APSED and the APT EID Programme was the extent to which the advances in outbreak detection and reporting for particular diseases would spread horizontally to improve detection and verification for other diseases or, conversely, the extent to which it drew resources and attention away from these other diseases. In the case of dengue, it is fair to argue that Japanese encephalitis has not experienced the reporting momentum seen for dengue because it is considered (for now) a mild disease without the same potential for reinfection—unlike dengue, which can develop into dengue hemorrhagic fever (although there remain those concerned the cases suspected to be Japanese encephalitis could mask more-deadly Nipah infections). Likewise, the reporting of cholera was sidelined by the revised IHR, but even prior to this, as figure 5.2 shows, the reporting incidence for cholera was sporadic at best in the region, with many states including Thailand and Malaysia reluctant to report a disease that could affect tourism, given cholera's association with seafood and drinking water (Mahapatra et al. 2014).

In the revised IHR, the IHR Category 1 list (Annex 2) of diseases that require immediate reporting to the WHO need have only one suspected outbreak to constitute a potential PHEIC. Diseases in this category include polio, smallpox, SARS, and any new human influenza strain. The H1N1 outbreak in 2009 fell into this category but was tabled as a respiratory infection for inclusion in this chapter, given the difficulty at the time in tracing reports of respiratory infection in the region that were specifically H1N1 in 2009 and 2010. In addition to H1N1, the region experienced SARS and H5N1 as IHR Category 1 outbreaks, and their specific reporting patterns for the region I have already discussed above. The only report under IHR Category 1 that was made, and of particular interest given the country, was the detection of two polio cases in Myanmar in 2007—which were officially reported (Myanmar was since declared officially polio-free in 2014).

By contrast, disease outbreaks under the IHR Category 2 list may not require immediate notification to the WHO unless the outbreak elicits two yes answers to one of the four questions in Annex 2. The diseases under the IHR Category 2 include cholera, pneumonic plague, yellow fever, viral hemorrhagic fevers (include Ebola, Lassa, and Marburg), West Nile fever, and other diseases of particular national concern (e.g., meningococcal disease or dengue fever). Within the ASEAN region, only one country has reported to the WHO a potential PHEIC under IHR 2—the Philippines experienced an outbreak of Ebola Reston fever in pig populations in Bulacan and Pangasinan Provinces between 2008 and 2009, with five farmers testing positive for the disease (but no symptoms). In these two cases (Myanmar with polio and the Philippines with Ebola), the promptness of the two governments—particularly Myanmar given its apparent reluctance to report disease outbreaks in general—indicates some awareness of the political ramifications of concealing outbreaks that require immediate notification under the IHR Annex 2.

A study on timeliness in disease reporting and preparedness by Richard Coker and colleagues (first in 2006, with a follow-up study in 2011) examined the performance of Southeast Asian states specifically concerning pandemic preparedness. Coker et al. noted in 2011 that the region had overall experienced a marked improvement in influenza reporting *and* response (verification). I too find that ASEAN states *overall* kept pace with the rate of SARS, H5N1, and respiratory outbreaks (including the 2009–2010 H1N1 outbreak). Official reports were issued to confirm outbreak events with increasing regularity. Informal reports tended to be the "suspected" reports—the reports of events unverified. Importantly, as figure 5.5 shows, few states over this period had informal reports of an outbreak event, such as H5N1, which was not followed up by the state with official confirmation. Myanmar, again, was the notable exception, with highest number of unverified reports across largest spread of diseases, followed by Cambodia, then Indonesia.

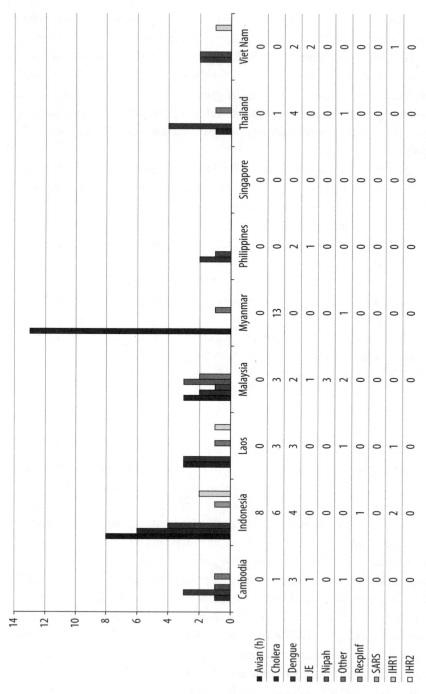

Figure 5.5. Informal Reports (by Disease Type) That Remained Unverified in ASEAN, 1996–2010

	Cambodia	Indonesia	Laos	Malaysia	Myanmar	Philippines	Singapore	Thailand	Viet Nam
■ Avian (h)	0	8	0	0	0	0	0	0	0
■ Cholera	1	6	3	3	13	0	0	1	0
■ Dengue	3	4	3	2	0	2	0	4	2
■ JE	1	0	0	1	0	1	0	0	2
■ Nipah	0	0	0	3	0	0	0	0	0
■ Other	1	0	1	2	1	0	0	1	0
■ RespInf	0	1	0	0	0	0	0	0	0
▨ SARS	0	0	0	0	0	0	0	0	0
□ IHR1	0	2	1	0	0	0	0	0	1
□ IHR2	0	0	0	0	0	0	0	0	0

One concern with the reporting trajectory is the region's continued difficulty in following up on the outbreaks that are not easily identified. This is particularly clear in the "other" reporting category in the dataset. Here, events were documented when the illness or deaths were not verified. The symptoms could range from unexplained diarrhea, respiratory illness, or rashes affecting a family or small community to news reports of unexpected deaths among a group of young individuals (including children) reported as being investigated by "health authorities," as well as reports that health authorities were investigating suspect outbreaks of enterovirus or meningococcal origin and the likelihood that the outbreak was infectious was high. Though these informal reports never reach above three per year for any country, their presence remains a persistent problem across the time span—one to two unverified diseases being informally reported but never followed up by an official source to confirm and verify. The state that had a persistent record for this during this time frame was Myanmar, with the highest number of unverified reports (striking given this country is more likely than others to have strict controls on media at the time), then Indonesia followed with a broader spread of different diseases being reported as suspected but not verified, followed by Cambodia.

The next chapter will discuss in more detail how we might interpret state-level reporting gaps as well as the different interpretations that states give to their own reporting obligations. What is clear is that diseases with political interest, funding programs, and media attention tend to have more official activity to detect and verify. However, it was not only the readily securitized outbreaks like H5N1 that received official attention. Regional political interest appears to be have been as deterministic an effect on what diseases received attention, as evidenced by the high volume of dengue outbreak reports, but it is also clear that the IHR have been formative in shaping states' detection and reporting practices. Even the most recalcitrant reporting state (i.e., Myanmar) predictably reported at some point during an outbreak that attracted regional concern. The outstanding problem is that endemic diseases without regional or WHO-level attention continue to go undetected. The role of the WHO in shaping reporting behavior in the region—via the IHR Annex 2—has the potential for great sway. It is the WHO's role and reporting practices in the region that I now examine.

The WHO Was Reporting EIDs

Over the 14-year period covered by this study, reporting to the WHO was steady but did not experience the rise in the same way that official state-level reporting overall increased (see figures 5.1 and 5.4). The highest peak in reports to the WHO came from Indonesia: 23 reports in 2006, while in the same year the Indonesian government officially communicated to the public 31 reports on outbreak events (mostly H5N1 human infections). The notable rise in WHO-issued reports from the region began in 2003 and concerned the SARS outbreak in Singapore and Viet Nam, and from 2005 to 2008, which specifically relate to the H5N1 infections in humans in Indonesia and Viet Nam. The two outbreaks were notified directly to the WHO, and the WHO was to post these events on *DON*, given their international concern. The question is whether the gap between the volume of reports the WHO listed on these outbreaks, particularly for Indonesia and Viet Nam, and the volume of state-issued reports on these same outbreaks during the same year indicates a problem in how outbreaks were being communicated to the WHO. (As noted, there was a difference between 23 WHO reports and 31 Indonesian government reports in 2006; the WHO's highest number of reports on H5N1 in Viet Nam was in 2005—it issued 12 reports against Viet Nam's 28.)

One point to note is a methodological one (which this study cannot answer without access to the WHO members-only Early Warning Management System): the volume of reports that *may* have been issued to the WHO by the state that WHO headquarters decided not to post on *DON*. Judgments can be made only with the data available, and there are two possible explanations for why reports received by the WHO were always fewer than state-issued reports on disease outbreak incidence in the ASEAN region.

The first explanation is that, in the early years of the revised IHR, reporting expectations to the WHO were undefined. The emphasis in these early years, communicated to the author by two donor-state officials who worked on the first APSED document, was placed squarely on enhancing regional discussion and transparency (Anonymous 2008a, 2011d). Similar views were expressed in interviews with WHO officials located in the Pacific and in at least three country offices in the WPRO and SEARO regions (ASEAN states) (Anonymous 2008d, 2010c, 2010g, 2010h, 2010k, 2010l, 2012g). In the early years of the IHR revisions, communicating to WHO headquarters was considered—by those in the region—less a priority than sharing outbreak events with the WPRO or SEARO via communicable disease sections. These regional sections then decided whether to notify WHO headquarters. The idea of states communicating with someone outside the state about an outbreak event (especially communicating that the Health Ministry could not yet verify what the outbreak was), rather than with WHO headquarters specifically, was seen as the crucial behavioral change, and this was what was to be emphasized under the first phase of APSED. Individuals associated with APSED's first phase said in interviews that IHR notification to headquarters was to be a rare event, a tool of last resort to compel states in the region to first report to SEARO or the WPRO. A WPRO official explained to the author that states preferred to report to the regional office, and this was emphasized to assist countries that were uncomfortable with the idea of reporting immediately to headquarters to feel comfortable reporting to *someone*: "IHR Annex 2 is not the best mechanism for encouraging reporting. IHR is to be avoided in most cases. The key is for WPRO to be part of states analysis of PHEIC. This is the key. So that IHR focal points in each country will rarely report up to WHO headquarters and not 'spook' everyone" (Anonymous 2008c).

The implication here was that, despite the revised IHR, states with low capacity for surveillance and verification remained wary about constantly reporting to WHO headquarters. In particular, they feared that a surplus of public reports of "unknown" outbreaks would create significant bureaucratic burdens and public panic that could result in economic uncertainty. To encourage reporting and transparency, the WPRO and SEARO presented themselves as mediators between the state and headquarters—working in cooperation with ministries on what to report to WHO headquarters and what to communicate only through the Ministry of Health. This was relayed to the author in different contexts, but one striking example of how confident the region had become with its communication processes under APSED was when the Indonesian minister of health, Siti Fadilah Supari, threatened to no longer notify the WHO of H5N1 human outbreaks.

Supari at the time believed that her government was coming under too much criticism from WHO headquarters for refusing to share virus samples unless Indonesia received guarantees of affordable access to whatever vaccine and antivirals were developed from those samples (Supari 2008). A SEARO official explained that this political dispute did not undermine quiet cooperation at the regional level:

> In reality, WHO Indonesia Country Office continued to work very closely with Indonesian Ministry of Health. Indonesian Ministry of Health worked very closely with WHO country office. WHO country office was informed of outbreaks. Sometimes these reports were informal and WHO country office were asked not to formally report further. We would wait to see if [the] outbreak was confirmed, if it was we would report to SEARO, who would report to headquarters. Even

those informal alerts would be sent to SEARO and headquarters—but we would ask to keep them quiet. This was all about timely response. We wanted feedback, we wanted trust. We knew so no need to alert [go public]. (Anonymous 2010m)

This point was understood at WHO headquarters in Geneva. An official there at the time expressed the view that they understood the position Indonesia had to publicly adopt because access to affordable vaccines and drugs was probably only going to be achieved "*this way*. So we trusted our regional counterparts to keep us informed" (Anonymous 2007b). In other words, despite the public political confrontation, WHO headquarters had sufficient confidence that, should the outbreak intensify in human-to-human transmission, the SEARO system would communicate with headquarters. Trust within the WHO system was more important than public communication of outbreak events at the time.

The second explanation for the gap between official reporting and WHO reporting is that WHO headquarters, WHO regional offices, and the state had different interpretations of when to report even on the same outbreaks. WHO regional offices developed their own practice for relaying disease outbreaks to WHO headquarters (only in the situations when the state had not already notified WHO headquarters itself). In the immediate aftermath of the adoption of the IHR revisions, the regional role in deciding which reports to communicate to Geneva appeared to be encouraged. Because reporting and verification procedures under APSED were presented as having the same thresholds as detailed in the IHR—24-hour time frame, the capacity to verify a suspected outbreak and request external assistance to verify whether national capacity was lacking—there was confidence that this would avoid regional offices sitting on events that could, in the words of a Geneva-based WHO official, "go wrong." Speaking specifically of SARS, this same official maintained that the WPRO regional office had been "caught off guard, and they won't wait for this to happen again" (Anonymous 2007b). This view was corroborated by an alert and response official at WHO headquarters who said that the real agenda of the revised IHR was to build *regional* capacity to assist states with joint assessment exercises (of risk of outbreak spread). After the experience of SARS and H5N1, the WHO had "no concerns" about the WPRO (and to "some extent" SEARO) carrying out joint risk assessments of outbreak situations (with the affected country) without headquarters (Anonymous 2007a).

Seven years later, the Ebola outbreak in West Africa in 2014 and criticism of the WHO's failure to meet to discuss a PHEIC during the first six months of the outbreak prompted sharp criticism of AFRO for failing to relay the full volume of Ebola reports to headquarters. After independent reviews and at the insistence of key donor states, in 2016 the WHA passed Health Emergencies Resolution 69/30 (WHA69/30 2016), which required states to immediately notify WHO headquarters of a disease outbreak event. WHO regional offices may be notified at the same time but would no longer be the only recipient of outbreak information. The 2016 Resolution establishes a potentially deep fault line within the system, since at the time of the adoption of the revised IHR, the WPRO and SEARO were quite strident on the need for states to have the option to report to the regional office rather than to headquarters. In the interviews for this book, the majority of which were conducted between 2007 and 2012, it is this regional dimension that has been identified as effective in the Southeast Asian case.

On balance, understanding how assessment and reporting is managed in practice goes a long way toward explaining the difference in WHO reports on *DON* on outbreak events in the region, compared with state-issued reports for the same outbreaks. Interviews with WHO headquarters officials tended to expose strong support for WHO country offices and the view that regional offices should be a conduit in relaying messages on outbreaks prior to communicating them to headquarters, rather than headquarters having to sift through and manage the "political, economic, and cultural relationships and repercussions of every event in each state" (Anonymous 2007a).

It is important to separate out the WHO's presence in the region and its role required in the reporting process. The publicly available data shows that WHO headquarters only sought to provide public notice of outbreak events in Southeast Asia for high-profile emerging infectious disease outbreaks like H5N1, SARS, and the diseases that came under the IHR Annex 2 Category 1 and Category 2 list—in other words, outbreak events deemed of international concern that may affect travel and trade. Outside of these events, WHO headquarters relied upon health ministries, WHO country offices (if present in the country), and WHO regional offices. These other actors were delegated the role of judging the soundness of the reports they were receiving. Whom to approach when surveillance and detection was absent, was a political judgment to be made between WHO regional office and WHO headquarters only after technical relationships had been exhausted. This is why, in the case of Indonesia during the height of the H5N1 outbreak, there was no public alarm (compared to SARS) raised by WHO headquarters about Supari's threat to end the reporting of suspect H5N1 infections in humans in 2007. SEARO and WHO headquarters staff were confident their relationships with Indonesian Health Ministry would sustain communication channels—but it would be discrete and informal. Over the years the prevailing view was that a small delay in publicly reporting an outbreak (or no report at all) was preferable if it ensured that technical information was still available through the epistemic networks. This is precarious terrain to navigate. It is far from predictable and can go wrong, as the Ebola outbreak in West Africa demonstrated. In the case of Southeast Asia, navigating the politics of surveillance and response is what led to the invitation of ASEAN into the APSED framework.

In the case of APSED, regional institutions played a vital two-step role in merging the WHO goal of IHR compliance with states' interest in strengthening core capacities such as surveillance and response operations for the novel outbreaks *and* endemic diseases like dengue, in an effort to normalize risk communication between states. Regional bodies were familiar in structure and behavior, which in turn served to play a key role in enhancing communication and trust between the actors (ministry, WHO region, WHO headquarters) vital for that first state of disease outbreak detection and verification.

Conclusion

Disease surveillance emerged as a priority for Southeast Asia even prior to the IHR revisions, perhaps explaining in part why the region accepted the IHR revisions. That said, the IHR created an added impetus for reform and political engagement at the regional level (Heywood and Moussavi 2010). Event-based surveillance mechanisms have been identified as the primary enabler for controlling the outbreak of infectious disease because of their early warning function—when these systems are running at full speed, they monitor, evaluate, model, detect, and track with the ultimate goal of seeking to contain or at least limit the impact (Castillo-Salgado 2010).

Control of the outbreak message was one that ASEAN states quickly seized post-SARS, and it was an act that WHO regional offices and headquarters supported. States continued to report outbreak events promptly, even when experiencing high outbreak events during this phase, and this was different compared to other regions (Chan et al. 2010). Southeast Asian states appeared to be attempting to "outpace" reports from informal sources. Interest has been to cover not only the IHR Annex 2 diseases but also those of regional concern that have not always made it onto the global agenda—particularly dengue. This was a region that evidently grasped the need to conduct surveillance and reporting, and to communicate competence in this area to local populations and neighboring states. Overall, the pattern of outbreak reports in the region over time demonstrates that receptiveness to the surveillance project requires not just technical and financial capacity but political will.

The regional trend for reporting improved over time, particularly during the first phase of APSED, but individual states' progress varies considerably. How to make sense of states' varied reporting trends is the subject of the next chapter. There I will show that the trend toward enhanced detection and reporting is at most risk in two areas: follow-up verification of initial disease outbreak reports and confronting the political situations that affect state capacity to detect and respond.

CHAPTER SIX

Understanding the Differences in Reporting Responsibilities

Why do states internalize their reporting responsibilities differently? As the previous chapter illustrated, Southeast Asia as a whole exhibited stronger compliance with the IHR's reporting requirements, with increased formal reporting widely evident. However, the chapter also identified some significant variations across diseases and countries. For those diseases that were specifically attached to the IHR or that had particular regional significance (e.g., SARS, H5N1, and dengue), we saw attempts by officials to outpace informal reports and deliver news on events to the community, to neighboring states, and to the WHO. Some of the states most affected by these diseases also sought to strengthen their official capacity to report outbreak events: Indonesia and Viet Nam account for more than half of the avian influenza cases reported, and it was the health ministries in both countries that dominated the reporting sources. Indonesia and Viet Nam dedicated significant political attention and material resources to H5N1 reporting. Given that H5N1 was of regional and international significance, this makes sense. However, in these same countries the record of reporting other diseases was significantly lower despite the fact that they experienced endemic outbreaks of possibly greater scale than H5N1 (dengue is a good example for both countries). In contrast, countries such as Myanmar, Cambodia, and Laos had few outbreak reports of any kind. Myanmar had more informal reports than official, while Cambodia and Laos had barely any informal reports.

How do we make sense of the individual cases that differ from the regional trends? Given the importance of sharing knowledge of outbreak events under the revised IHR, a revision that was endorsed by the Southeast Asian region in APSED and ASEAN statements, when does an individual failure indicate a more systemic problem? And, where we see systemic problems, how do we know whether to attribute these to shortfalls in health system capacity, as opposed to shortfalls of political will?

In this chapter, I address these questions by examining two critical conditions that impact upon the performance of health systems in the detection and verification process: the country's political system and the capacity of its health system. I argue that the different demands that diseases place on national health capacity as well as the political context in which a disease outbreak or disease event emerges tells us that factors *other than* the general level of commitment to early warning surveillance and reporting play a significant role in shaping reporting behavior in individual country cases.

The Political Will to Report: Variation across States

The WHO (2017g: 22) has recently acknowledged the relationship between good governance and transparent reporting, and the need for (politically) safe conditions to report:

> Notably, public health professionals themselves sometimes require protection. As champions of the common good, they must be free to report without fear of reprisal. As surveillance officials have a responsibility to speak up, they should have protection. This idea is established in the IHR, which protects the confidentiality of those who report a verifiable outbreak or a public health event outside official channels. (35)

As discussed in chapter 1, a significant shift within the revised IHR was that states agreed to openly and promptly report outbreaks with the *potential* for international spread (Li and Kasai 2011: 7). This agreement led to the idea that states appoint an IHR National Focal Point to be available 24/7 in every country to communicate outbreak events with the WHO. Michael Baker and David Fidler (2006) argue that an additional important inclusion under the revised IHR was the provision that gave the WHO the right to receive reports of disease outbreak events *from sources other than the affected state*: Article 9—Other Reports. Specifically, Article 9 permits the WHO to "take into account reports [of outbreak events] from sources other than notifications or consultations and shall assess these reports according to established epidemiological principles and then communicate information on the event to the State Party in whose territory the event is allegedly occurring" (WHO 2008: Article 9). The article also refers to the following: "Only where it is duly justified may WHO maintain the confidentiality of the source" (9.1). Article 9 permits the WHO to receive reports of disease outbreaks from sources other than the state and for the WHO to exercise its own judgment on protecting the confidentiality of that source.

In practice, the right of the WHO to receive reports from informants other than the state on outbreak events and to protect the identity of those informants is difficult to actualize (S. Davies 2017). The reality is that some states remain able and willing to ensure that this right not be exercised. The balance to be struck in this region and others is the state's need to manage risk communication to prevent panic and misinformation against the citizens' right to information, and the non-state actors' right to report outbreak information. Article 9 within the revised IHR provides for the right of non-state actors to report to the WHO, but there is no corresponding framework in international human rights law relating to how this right may be enacted. In the initial stages there are few means available to determine what the absence of reporting means or why a state may fail to correct or address a non-state report. Unless an instance of arrest and intimidation occurs (Madoff and Woodall 2005), is a state deliberately withholding outbreak information, or does the state "just" not know the full extent of an outbreak because it lacks the health system capacity to detect or verify an outbreak? There is no perfect means of deducing when political interference in the reporting process, rather than a poorly functioning health system, is affecting the pace and flow of reports. However, there are patterns that suggest some states are more inclined to regularly exert political pressure on the surveillance and response system than other states.

By virtue of the confidentiality clause, there is little public information about when the WHO has protected the identity of an informal reporter to secure news of an outbreak event. My study of reports in chapter 5 shows that in Southeast Asia, Viet Nam, Indonesia, Thailand, Malaysia, Philippines, and Singapore have the highest concentration of official confirmations over this period (in order). Myanmar, Laos, and Cambodia have the lowest official confirmations. However, some of these same countries—Indonesia and Malaysia—also have some of the highest rates of informal (non-state report) confirmations. In contrast, Cambodia and Myanmar stand out (figure 6.1) for having informal reports that outnumber (Myanmar) or equal (Cambodia) their release of official reports, while Singapore, Laos, and Viet Nam have the lowest number of informal reports over this period (in order).

How should we interpret these practices against the expected conditions on the freedom to report? Does a high number of informal reports that have not been verified reveal inadequate attention to outbreaks by the government? Conversely, is a low number of informal reports evidence of a government that is placing limits on media reporting or of a coordinated risk communication strategy between government and media? The IHR (2005) are underpinned by Article 3.1, which states, "The implementation of these Regulations shall be with full respect for the dignity, human rights and fundamental freedoms of persons" (WHO 2008). This was the first time the IHR had referred to a

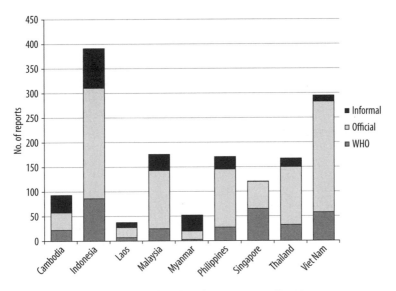

Figure 6.1. Total Source of Outbreak Reports in ASEAN, 1996–2010

relationship between human rights and containment of disease outbreaks. After the political interference in reporting infections and deaths due to SARS in China, but also experiences prior to China of political resistance to the WHO receiving and communicating outbreak reports (Fidler 2004b), the inclusion of human rights in the revised IHR signaled to "governments worldwide that their obligations to their citizens (as well as those temporarily within their borders) extend[ed] into all realms—including public health and infectious disease control" (Youde 2009: 167).

To date, most discussion on the human rights provisions within the IHR have referred to the freedom of the (infected and noninfected) individual to move freely and travel during disease outbreaks (Plotkin 2007). However, civil and political rights conditions in an affected country may also influence and determine the WHO's access to information and non-state actors' right to report in an emergency situation (WHO 2017g). If Article 9 is to be fully realized by non-state actors—whether media, NGOs, or individuals—who report in defiance of their government, the IHR must have a much broader human rights dimension. How essential is the right to report to the relationship between positive fulfilment of civil and political rights for outbreak surveillance and response?[1] The WHO has to balance its potential need for non-state reports with the need for state cooperation and public trust in the emergency response of the state (38). How much does this right to report need to be considered when tracing what reforms states are engaging in to be IHR compliant?

One way to measure the promptness and transparency of the process from detection to verification is to trace when a report (by any source) is first made, when the relevant state has been first notified of an outbreak, the date of public notice of laboratory confirmation, and the date of public communication of the outbreak event (Chan et al. 2010: 5). Among the findings of one such study, Chan et al. (2010) found that the greatest risk of a public information delay was between first detection of an outbreak and public communication of an outbreak. Delays occurred when governments decided to publicly communicate only after laboratory confirmation. The potential for conflict between official and nonofficial sources comes at this moment—the point at which there is information, as yet unverified, of a potential outbreak. At this stage, concerned individuals may seek to report their findings, their suspicions, or their evidence while the state is waiting for confirmation, sometimes to force the state to quicken its own procedures. Delaying communication carries two risks. First, if the outbreak is serious and the state does not have the laboratory capacity to detect, crucial containment time may be lost. Second, the information vacuum may diminish the trust of those most being affected by the outbreak in their government, prompting them to seek information from alternative sources and to resist information finally relayed by formal sources. This can allow misinformation to flourish and make it more difficult for governments to conduct effective risk communication. Yet there are also reasons to delay communication until after verification.

Reporting only laboratory-confirmed outbreaks minimizes public panic. It was often remarked that reports of suspected cases were something the sensationalist media did, and when that happened it was against the wishes of the state. There was also a concern that the regular release of suspect reports could undermine trust in risk communication. The view that communication should be delayed until verification was a common one that I encountered in interviews right across the region, but especially in the Mekong region. Traced over time some governments, such as Cambodia and Viet Nam, have increasingly publicly notified suspect outbreaks, but often the government notices appeared very close to the same time that the government provided laboratory confirmation. In the case of Cambodia, the country has consistently reported failure to reach 100% for most of the IHR core capacities (see table 6.1 and chap. 1), and this undoubtedly affected its official reporting practices (see figure 6.1).

In 2010, Myanmar reported 100% compliance across the IHR core capacities (see table 6.1 on p. 154 and chap. 1) but during the phase examined had more informal reports on outbreak events and rarely provided official outbreak communication reports (only in the later years and mostly on a notifiable disease established to be in the region, i.e., H1N1). In contrast with Cambodia, which does not claim to have 100% capacity, the Myanmar government may either be regarded as not having the IHR capacity that it claims or as having that capacity but choosing not to officially inform its public and neighboring states of outbreak events. If it is the latter, then the presence of informal media reports in Myanmar during this period is all the more curious. Either these were genuine informal reports that managed to detect and report outbreak events without the government's consent (and, note, there was no official follow-up to the informal reports), or the "informal" reports were actually issued by the media with government consent. The point here is that differentiating between capacity and government interference when it comes to reporting is a difficult task; it carries risk for the WHO when it acts on an informal report, in particular; and the norm of officially communicating laboratory-confirmed outbreaks is a behavior borne of states that fear being unable to manage the consequences of earlier disclosure of suspect outbreak events.

In interviews government officials across the region repeatedly suggested that the media and government had an informal understanding that the media should not report suspected outbreaks without permission from the Ministry of Health. This was, again, particularly strong in the Mekong region. There is no formal regulation or legislation that sets out this understanding, but it is one that the media and private laboratories are aware of and know they must abide by to remain informed "friends" of the ministry. As Kluberg and colleagues (2016) argue, it is these region-specific customs and behavior that shed light on what obstacles remain to progressing surveillance and response. These practices are difficult to capture in self-report surveys of IHR compliance and ones that few states will own to in external evaluation exercises because of their informal nature. But no one doubts it occurs and it has influence on the speed of outbreak detection and containment. Political interference in the process for detection to verification and then communication can create moments of intense uncertainty and risk, and delays in response. How do you gain trust and cooperation from a regime that does not trust its own population, and how do neighboring states trust the regime in turn? One subtle answer to this concern in the first phase of APSED was risk communication.

Risk communication in the region has primarily focused on how states should manage the public communication of an outbreak event. The first phase of APSED established the idea under the fifth program that risk communication was the public deserving to know and receive the facts from official sources sooner than later (WPRO 2012). In the Philippines, Indonesia, and to some extent Thailand, I observed much discussion on risk communication that focused on how to manage the flow of informal reports that were often incorrect and were determined to provoke fear (and, from that, generate readership) and on the frustration of local officials contradicting federal ministry communication instructions—in other words, the type of risk communication management concerns familiar to democratic governments experiencing high(er) rates of informal and official reports throughout the period studied. Officials often also expressed concern about decisions to report or not in conditions (nearly universal across Southeast Asia) where prior executive approval to communicate was essential. In public, the practice of reporting is rarely connected to discussions on governance, transparency, and civil liberties. Yet, in private, these underlying conditions for risk communication are often acknowledged, but raising transparency and civil liberties to improve communication was a step too far in the public forums. This meant that the confidentiality provision in Article 9, for example, was often presented in APSED workshops as "report first or you will be beaten by the rumors." The example of Singapore—an autocratic regime with fairly rigid censorship controls providing a positive risk communication strategy—was often used to illustrate how reporting could be done: it managed SARS with daily official communication, a centralized message, and a 24-hour patient trace system (Bennett 2009: 53; WPRO 2012). Of course, Singapore is a unique city-state and its experiences are not readily transferrable, but it is the broader strategy that is of interest here: the attempt by an authoritarian state to grant transparency "lite" in order to meet the demands of risk communication without sacrificing broader control. This practice contrasts to the preference that APSED (and the ASEAN secretariat) were trying to address among a number of states: to control the message during the early stages of outbreak emergencies in case the media reports the information. Therefore, it is no surprise that concerted effort and investment in risk communication was again repeated in Phase 2 (2010–2015) of the APSED program.

The question is the sustainability of this strategy and what happens when the message to report early and report often goes awry in a situation where the state has connected political survival to secrecy. We generally understand that civil and political freedoms tend to improve disease outbreak reporting conditions, so we should also expect to see informal reports increase (e.g., Brownstein et al. 2008; Chan et al. 2010; S. Davies 2012). In other words, the risk of outbreak is managed by a communication chain that does not attempt to prevent informal reports but is promptly responded to by official channels to reassure the public and ensure the most scientifically accurate measure if relayed (O'Malley, Rainford, and Thompson 2009). The expectation has been that informal reports of disease outbreaks will increase as internet surveillance and biosurveillance capacity is enhanced with greater use of internet and technological devices among the populace. Yet this is not happening in Southeast Asia. Few countries, perhaps including Indonesia and Philippines, with Thailand and Malaysia coming in a distant third and fourth, have a strong informal reporting sector across the disease types. Non-state actors have limited means with which to report a message that is different from the state's.

The campaign for including a right for the WHO to receive media and other sources of outbreak reports under the revised IHR was based on the argument that such information will come out whether states like it or not (Fidler 2004b). Therefore, the argument goes, informal reports can be used to the international community's advantage, whether by prompting states to report themselves in the expectation that if they do not, someone else will, or simply by improving the WHO's situational awareness (Heymann and Rodier 2005). At the same time, it has been pointed out that informal reporting depends upon transparent and risk-free communication opportunities in countries (S. Davies 2012). In other words, reports are more likely to emerge from those states with liberal reporting and civil rights; individuals who report from countries with restricted reporting and civil rights, as well as limited open internet access, risk attracting penalties and will therefore likely be deterred (Rod and Weildman 2015). This is not occurring in most countries in Southeast Asia. In countries such as Cambodia, Laos, Myanmar, and Viet Nam, however, where there is a recent history of repression of journalists and strong censorship laws, the risk is always present that there will be political interference with public health risk communication.

As I have shown, information control coupled with the need for governments to be responsive to regional health security threats has encouraged government communication to become faster and more public. The APSED framework and the APT EID plans have certainly encouraged this activity. But can this control create perverse risks and incentives to avoid detection? In the case of Viet Nam, Jonathan Herrington (2010) points out that the government response to the H5N1 outbreak—forced poultry culling and small compensation for the loss of livelihood—led to farmers seeking to hide poultry and outbreaks. It was not the state hiding outbreak events but local populations fearful of loss of income. In the same country, HIV status is no longer a "social evil" according to government policy, but the two groups at most risk of HIV infection—prostitutes and drug users—suffer from negative social stereotypes. In situations where the political response to a disease outbreak may be discriminatory, it may be harsh, it may lack empathic response, and it may promote social stigma, the conditions necessary to achieve prompt and effective surveillance and response will be difficult.

When we are attempting to track the efficiency and coverage of surveillance from detection to reporting to verification—at the national or regional level—we need to pay greater attention to the political systems in which surveillance operates. The WHO and surveillance sites like ProMED may be in a position to receive non-state reports but be in no situation to protect the human rights of those who take the risk to report and face punishment from the state for such reporting (WHO 2011). The expectation has been that Article 9 will compel states to improve their own surveillance and reporting practices to beat non-state actors and neighboring states that may report under Article 9. An alternative view is that Article 9 drives states to be more secretive—and to exercise control over freedom of information exchange among those in the health sector, in the media, and in civil society. The success of the IHR requires political transparency as much as it requires technical proficiency in surveillance and response, but how to protect those who wish to report in situations where governments resist the transparency that is forced upon them with a 24/7 surveillance and response system? In chapters 4 and 5, I argued that APSED achieved political traction because of its deliberate engagement of regional institutions like ASEAN and APT. States are the primary actors being appealed to and supported in building their capacity (Heywood and Moussavi 2010). Where the APSED and ASEAN secretariat struggled in the first phase is confronting and discussing the situation where a state may be in control of the message, may be in control of the verification process, and still seek to block reports from media, civil society, or public health officials that contradict the state's message.

The UN secretary-general-appointed High Level Panel on the Global Response to Health Crises, released in early 2016, came closest to addressing this issue when it referred to efforts by some governments to downplay the extent of the Ebola outbreak in their country by calling (international) NGOs "alarmist" (High Level Panel 2016). The panel noted that the governments where there was dysfunction and secrecy had the least familiarity with conducting public information campaigns to empower populations and challenge rumors. Familiarity with transparency, the panel found, was essential to build health capacity—to enhance preparedness, response, and communication during outbreaks.

In executing IHR compliance, the freedoms and transparency afforded under a political regime is significant; the freedom in which civil society, media, and health care workers can exchange information easily is essential. We cannot definitely point to every situation where there was a reporting gap between detection and verification as the result of politicization, especially in a country that also has substandard health system capacity to detect and respond. However, this is the challenge for IHR reform—how to sensitively and inclusively manage political systems that can be responsive to the capacity changes required. No technical system can avoid the social and political changes that also need to accompany risk communication. In the ASEAN case, the consistent argument has been that the importance of regional engagement and cooperation is its creation of a diplomatically "safe space" to begin engaging in individual states' responsibility to provide safe conditions for reporting and communicating disease outbreak events. The risk remains that a state will seek to cover up an outbreak, and the best preemption of that risk to date in the ASEAN region has been more engagement, not less.

Health Systems Capacity

Not all points of variation have to do with the political system, however. Health systems capacity also impacts significantly on performance. How then to manage situations where the capacity to detect and verify may be compromised not by politics but by competing public health priorities (Coker et al. 2011)? One thing that is clear is that different understandings persist among states about (1) the order of the detection and reporting process and (2) what should be promptly reported (Chan et al. 2010: 4; Gostin and Freidman 2015). If we look at the 2010 self-reporting data ASEAN states provided to the WHO on their IHR core capacity compliance, we see some explanation for varied reporting practices that points to varied capacity and different understandings of which capacities should be prioritized.[2]

As discussed previously, the eight core capacity categories were legislation, coordination, surveillance, response, preparedness, risk communication, human

TABLE 6.1. ASEAN 2010 IHR Core Capacities

Country	Legisn	Coord	Surv	Resp	Prepare	Risk com	HR	Lab
Brunei	0	66	61	90	39	70	16	65
Cambodia	100	58	84	58	0	30	16	76
Indonesia	100	100	56	89	71	80	83	100
Laos	75	75	64	94	73	20	66	61
Malaysia	100	100	64	100	100	70	100	77
Myanmar	100	66	88	100	66	90	33	70
Philippines	0	48	88	58	66	90	33	80
Singapore	100	100	100	100	100	100	100	100
Thailand	50	100	52	94	73	50	66	83
Viet Nam	50	71	51	100	35	70	66	94

Source: WHO 2017a.

resources, and laboratory readiness. States could report their compliance within the following ranges from 0%–24%, 25%–49%, 50%–74%, to 75%–100%. ASEAN states self-reported the results shown in table 6.1.

The one capacity that all states self-reported as having the highest level of readiness was response (8 states reported in the 75%–100% category) followed by laboratory (7 states reported in the 75%–100% category) and risk communication (7 states again reported in the 75%–100% category). This was followed by legislation (6 out of 10 states reported themselves as being 75%–100% compliant) followed by 4 states reporting 75%–100% compliance in coordination and surveillance (remaining 6 reported themselves in the 50%–74% category), followed by preparedness and human resources at the least stages of readiness. This is, in many respects, an outcome that juxtaposes what the APSED focused on to what it presumed by the end of 2010. Surveillance, the necessary condition for response, did comparatively worse; states' sense of their ability to do risk communication was stronger than what, perhaps, those watching these states believed them to be. Moreover, it may be suggested there are some contradictions in these self-reports. Can states have such high capacity in their laboratory readiness when they report so low in the areas of surveillance and preparedness? If coordination and legislation are not yet reformed to meet the capacity benchmarks, how can states be so advanced with their risk communication and response procedures? Finally, given the low scores for human resources, it might be asked precisely who is meeting all these capacity targets? These apparent contradictions in how states judge their capacity readiness is even more apparent when we look at their individual scores, and it possibly points to two statements about the IHR in ASEAN at this stage in 2010. States comprehended the IHR as important and did not want to expose (at the domestic or international level) their lack of readiness (the glaringly obvious case here is Myanmar). The second point is that the self-reporting function allowed states to report on what they were comfortable reporting on and that states took to this task to either report poor readiness to demonstrate the need for continued donor investment (for example, Cambodia and Laos), or they reported fairly accurately where they believed they could meet expectations.

Curiously, given its focus in the APSED and APT EID, all countries with the exception of Singapore reported their surveillance readiness to be below full compliance. Cambodia, Myanmar, and Philippines reported capacity just below 100%, while Brunei, Indonesia, Laos, and Malaysia reported as being a little more than halfway compliant; Thailand and Viet Nam reported as being midway to achieving full compliance. If we compare these self-report assessments from 2010 with the progress in surveillance detection presented earlier, however, there are consistencies in how states perceive their performance against their actual performance (two notable exceptions being Cambodia and Myanmar).

Singapore's capacity to conduct surveillance and report is state directed but it has a consistent record of reporting outbreaks across the disease categories and, in the case of SARS, was commended for its readiness to report infectious caseloads. The Philippines is also a consistent reporter of outbreak events at the official level, and there is a high number of informal reports from the Philippines, but they do not outnumber the official reports, which indicates some consistency in the official response to the reported rumors of outbreak events and reporting of laboratory-confirmed outbreak events. The self-reporting capacity of Cambodia and Myanmar does not fit the picture of readiness both countries presented. Despite claiming to have the necessary capacity, neither state was among the region's best performers. That said, Cambodia in particular did begin to show consistent improvement in reporting capacity between 2005 and 2010, while Myanmar showed some signs of improved performance after 2009.

At the same time, surveillance performance differed across different diseases within the same country. Differences with respect to the reporting of respiratory illnesses were often explained by reference to geography and the bureaucratic systems. Interviews in countries with relatively weak health systems, such as Cambodia and Laos, and in those such as Thailand and Malaysia, where systems were much stronger, differences in reporting were explained as the inevitable result of different patterns of spread and reporting in provincial locations. Sometimes, reporting differences can be ascribed to the level of resources assigned to different diseases within the same country. Indonesia's reports on dengue, repeatedly prioritized in ASEAN joint statements on health matters, were lower than that of Cambodia. Yet it would be fairly safe to assume that dengue numbers would be higher in Indonesia than in Cambodia because of demographic and geographic factors alone. Yet resourcing decisions meant that Indonesia prioritized other health threats—including the threat posed by H5N1 and H1N1—over and above the risks posed by dengue, affecting patterns of reporting.

What then of the additional core capacities necessary to support and complement the conduct of surveillance? Legislative reform and the creation of a national coordinating focal point are capacities directed at supporting the reporting and containment process. These capacities are intended to serve in designating responsibility for reporting, receiving reports, and acting on reports. Human resourcing is then necessary to conduct the surveillance: individuals to fill the National Focal Point post, ensuring staff is available for surveillance, response, and coordination. The relationship among surveillance, response, and laboratory readiness to diagnose an outbreak also requires a preparedness plan to be in place, practiced, and ready for immediate implementation.

Laboratory readiness for most countries, except Indonesia and Singapore, was self-reported to be at between 75% and 100% of the required levels. Myanmar was only starting to emerge from a decades-long exile from the international community in 2010, yet it reported its laboratory capacity as 70%—similar (albeit marginally lower) to that of Malaysia and Thailand who reported (respectively) 77% and 83%. Cambodia reported 100% in legislative reform to meet the IHR capacity but provided no entry score for its preparedness capacity and reported its coordination capacity at 58%. Indonesia reported its surveillance capacity at 56%, its capacity to respond at 89%, and 71% preparedness capacity. Myanmar again claimed 100% capacity to respond, while the Philippines reported 58% response capacity, as did Cambodia. Cambodia and Laos reported, respectively, 30% and 20% capacity to conduct risk communication, while Myanmar and Philippines reported 90% capacity. Only Singapore claimed 100% capacity.

There is no baseline data to compare these reports against. These 2010 scores are the baseline for future assessments of states' progress in each of the eight core capacities. The claim to be 100% compliant requires states to deliver on what they report. But at the same time few presume that states such as Myanmar, in reporting 100% capacity, actually have this capacity. This then brings us back to the politics. Capacity assessments of technical proficiency, coordination, and preparedness are all political statements about the efficiency and stability of the regime. It is this combination of politics and capacity that has led to self-reporting practices under the IHR—and APSED—revealing a contradictory story for some states. Are there grounds to question the self-reporting capacity of states to the WHO in 2010, and how do we differentiate between ambition and capacity? Answering this question is vital if donor and political investment is to be made in regional arrangements to assist with IHR compliance.

The adoption of the IHR revisions coupled with the APSED programming arguably kept ASEAN states conscious of the standard they were expected to meet by 2012. As one Ministry of Health official from an ASEAN country said in an interview on laboratory preparedness, "You should never underestimate how competitive we ASEAN countries are. No one wants to show up at a workshop and say they have not progressed" (Anonymous 2012f). On the one hand, states want to impress each other with their progress, yet, on the other hand, there is the need to provide the opportunity to acknowledge and address different capacity standards. As one Ministry of Health official from a country in the Mekong Basin said, "Different countries have different domestic processes for reporting" (Anonymous 2010g). The same official went on to note that while *they* don't need the prime minister's approval for each alert on a H5N1 sample, officials in other neighboring countries were not in the same situation to report so freely. Likewise, few ministry officials can honestly report their structural and institutional deficiencies without professional consequences. In situations where health systems are already struggling, it may be safely assumed they will struggle to communicate outbreak events consistently and across a broad spectrum of diseases—despite what a state may report in terms of its IHR capacities.

What then is the use of the IHR reporting mechanism? It drives ASEAN states' behavior. As Richard Coker and colleagues (2011) note, there is now reasonable confidence that most ASEAN states can detect a H5N1 human infection case, but they cannot yet detect all Japanese encephalitis. This illustrates the tension identified in the APSED review (2010): the regional approach to building IHR core capacity yielded significant benefits but at the risk of allowing some states to avoid being confronted with their individual capacity shortfalls (particularly in environments where self-reporting was the norm for tracking capacity and proficiency). The self-reporting scores for IHR core capacities in 2010 clearly reveal this tension, with some countries giving themselves performance scores that are not an accurate depiction of their capacity. How then to identify the countries that require this engagement in a context where they may be politically resistant to exposing their incapacity? I maintain that, whatever their limitations, regional political institutions continue to play a vital role in bridging the gap between the global and the local, between the ambitions of WHO headquarters and the realities on the ground in Southeast Asia. Relationships within programs like APSED and APT EID provide safe venues to hear and voice obstacles under a veil of relative confidentiality in a forum where states understand the political as well as the technical capacity hurdles.

Conclusion

From the adoption of the IHR in 2005 to the end of the first APSED phase in 2010, ASEAN member states sought to significantly improve their disease-reporting behaviors. Part of this journey had already begun before the adoption of the IHR, but after the IHR adoption, the growth of formal reporting outpaced the growth of informal reporting by a significant margin. States sought to significantly improve their capacity and communication in the detection and reporting of disease outbreaks. This focus was often biased, with attention devoted to those diseases designated by the international community as international public health threats (e.g., H5N1 infection in humans, SARS, and H1N1) at the expense of others (e.g., Japanese encephalitis) not so designated. However, this chapter has emphasized that variation among diseases and countries is more complex than this and relates to political systems, the political will to detect and verify outbreak events, the capacity to meet the IHR surveillance and response expectations, and the relationships among all these considerations. I have identified situations where the region continues to have reporting "black holes"—outbreaks that are known to occur but for which there is no surveillance record—and situations where there are disease outbreak rumors that are not officially confirmed or denied. In these situations, the combination of political interference and health system capacity shortfalls permits countries to risk avoiding formal communication. Despite the investment of APSED and APT in normalizing surveillance and response, a small number of states have remained consistent in the inconsistent practice of detection and verification.

This has led to two patterns of behavior: reporting performance as meeting the required benchmark to avoid further inquiry—despite obvious difficulties with detection and reporting (e.g., Myanmar); or, as with Cambodia and Laos, swinging between openness and secrecy. These states straddle wanting to report their genuine difficulties with IHR compliance (to address capacity shortfalls), but they are also reluctant to expose political and bureaucratic leadership (often the same thing) to critique. It may be assumed that the burdens of political interference and capacity shortfalls are experienced in many ASEAN states, but particular countries are presenting an extreme example of health system incapacity coupled with political sensitivity to document and report. This is illustrative of the political culture in which IHR reform takes place and how it can accentuate existing implementation burdens, like capacity shortfalls. It also illustrates why political forums and the socialization of shared experiences, shared failure, and shared problems is vital. These technical tasks of capacity building are taking place in political environments with political consequences; that is why the regional dimension is such an important part of the picture.

The central importance of the regional dimension, and in particular of the buy-in of the region's political institutions, is evidenced by the fact that, compared to other regions, Southeast Asia has made significant progress toward IHR compliance. The Southeast Asian region has had the misfortune of a substantial period prior to the adoption of revised IHR of familiarity with outbreaks to become responsive to health security language. But arguably so have other regions. In such politically sensitive locations, APSED and APT EID facilitated the creation of shared language and shared understanding of IHR implementation and its relationship to regional security as a way of persuading states to view the initiative as something that does more to complement national interests than to challenge them. This arrangement is not foolproof. As shown in this chapter, it can still fall hostage to capacity and politics. Yet a region committed to sovereignty and noninterference has not only accepted the principle of surveillance and reporting on infectious disease, it has also moved to adopt that principle into practice. That shift could not have occurred without the role played by regional actors and institutions. The question now is whether this is sustainable.

The Sustainability of Health Security in Southeast Asia

The introduction of the revised IHR marked a watershed in the politics and practice of health security, especially with respect to their provisions on disease surveillance and reporting. For the first time, states were required to report the outbreak of a wide range of diseases, and the WHO was entitled to utilize reports from non-state sources whenever it saw fit. For a region like Southeast Asia, whose international relations are prefaced on principles of sovereignty and noninterference, the IHR constitute a critical challenge. Understandably, questions have been raised and concerns expressed about the capacity and willingness of states, not just those in Southeast Asia, to comply with the revised IHR in practice. Indeed, this question has been subject to multiple reviews over the past decade. Things were made more acute by the sense of failure that surrounded responses to the Ebola outbreak in West Africa in 2014. Concerns about the world's lackluster performance produced a flurry of new political commitments to health security and, in turn, the IHR (McInnes and Mahler 2017). The revised IHR were marveled at for their scope and demands on states performance when they were adopted (Fidler 2005), but they soon came to be regarded as both too narrow and too demanding, particularly for states with weak health systems: "Attempts to strengthen IHR-mandated core capacities without considering broader national health sector strategies risk creating IHR 'silos,' and reinforcing redundancies in countries already strained by scarce resources and inadequate health workforces" (Katz and Fischer 2010: 14–15). States in regions such as Southeast Asia would be both unable (because of the capacity demands) and unwilling (because of their effects on sovereignty) to comply with the surveillance and reporting demands imposed by the revised IHR. Or so it was widely assumed.

In previous research (Davies, Kamradt-Scott, and Rushton 2015), I argued that the revised IHR began their life with tremendous good will from member states. This was true in Southeast Asia, where support for the IHR arose out of already existing support for the concept of health security and, perhaps more importantly, recognition of the risks to health security. However, 10 years after the IHR were adopted, only a third of all states had achieved full compliance with the eight core capacities they demanded. This further fed doubts about whether the ambitious targets set by the IHR were ever possible, financially, politically, and logistically. Concerns arose that even some of those states that claimed to be in compliance with the regulations were in fact not in compliance at all. Meanwhile, others question whether the impetus to achieve the formally agreed upon goals would draw attention and resources away from the broader agenda of health systems strengthening, producing a hierarchy of illnesses in international relations that would determine the level of care provided (Enemark 2017).

With its conservative attitude toward sovereignty and noninterference, its relatively weak health systems, and its proclivity for new diseases, one would expect that Southeast Asia would be a particularly hard case for the revised IHR. Indeed, in the preceding pages I have demonstrated that the challenges faced by the region are legion. Yet, for all that, when it comes to the reporting of infectious disease, Southeast Asian states have demonstrated a consistently improved rate of compliance with the IHR, one that starkly contradicts claims that the IHR are a failed experiment in global health governance. Crucial to understanding *why* the region has achieved this is grasping that implementation of IHR is dependent not just on health systems themselves but also on the political regimes and regional contexts they occupy (International Working Group on Financial Preparedness 2017: 69; Moore et al. 2016). The technical functions demanded within the IHR do not exist in a political or institutional vacuum, however much some medical and public health actors wish this was the case. What is technical, what is public health, what is a risk, and what is an executive function are all potential sites of political contestation provoked by the IHR and their implementation. To understand why states comply, or do not comply, with the IHR, we need to understand their political, institutional, and material contexts and how the politics of health relates to the broader political context.

When we do that, we can begin to understand why Southeast Asia has exceeded global expectations when it comes to the reporting of infectious disease outbreaks. The answer lies in the uniquely political way in which it has approached the problem. Southeast Asia is an extremely diverse region that includes widely varying political, social, and economic conditions, not only among states (compare wealthy Singapore with impoverished Laos) but also within them too (there are stark differences, for example, between metropolitan Jakarta and outlying islands in Indonesia). The core capacity requirements under the IHR, that states signed in 2005, contain little if any recognition of different contexts (Caballero-Anthony et al. 2015). Yet, despite the stark differences, Southeast Asia has been recognized as being responsive to the normative goals of the revised IHR: to detect and report a broad category of potential public health emergencies (Chan et al. 2010; Li 2013; Australian Government 2017). To understand precisely why the region proved so receptive to these developments, we need to understand what the region thought about global health prior to the emergence of the IHR and how it has gone about responding to the challenge of implementing them.

In chapter 3, I showed that, even prior to the development of the IHR, Southeast Asian governments had come to embrace the concept of health security—a phrase that was strongly attached to the IHR at the time of the revision negotiation. Indeed, by the time that the international community came together on the IHR, most Southeast Asian governments had already incorporated a concept of health security into their understandings of national security and had also recognized the important regional dynamic—namely, that security from infectious disease could not be achieved by any single state: it required action by the whole region. This recognition explains why sovereignty has not blocked the IHR in Southeast Asia. To understand why the region so readily accepted the view that infectious disease was a transnational threat that required a transnational response, we need look no further that the region's own recent experience. The shared experiences of the Nipah, SARS, and then H5N1 outbreaks in quick succession, and especially the political, economic, and social upheavals that these outbreaks risked creating, dispelled the notion that traditional approaches to security, suffused with sovereignty and noninterference, would be sufficient. These experiences taught states that no amount of health systems capacity (e.g., Singapore) or tightly managed political order (e.g., Viet Nam) could protect societies from infectious disease. States would remain vulnerable if they continued to frame their response only in national terms. Lived experience brought the region's states to this understanding at precisely the same time that this narrative was being promoted by the WHO. This convergence of views, between the region and the WHO, spurred the creation of APSED in 2005: a program that networked member states from two WHO regions—Western Pacific and South-East Asia—to commit to supporting one another in the provision of technical advice, workshops, and training in IHR compliance and regional health security. It was unlike anything the two WHO regions had attempted before—it was to be driven by the region itself, inclusive of regional needs and interests, and sensitive to the region's specific context and challenges. It was, in other words, led by the region itself. These conditions were vital in its early days of trial and tribulation.

APSED effectively made the IHR a regional project. Between 2005 and 2010, APSED consistently positioned itself as a collective regional effort to meet the region's own challenges by implementing the IHR in a way that corresponded with the region's interests and sensitivities. Meeting the core capacities was not "just" a requirement under international law, something demanded by outsiders or imposed from above. Instead, it was understood to be of immense benefit and importance for the health of the region, the economy of the region, and the political security of the region. Within this context, most ASEAN states—even the capacity poor (Cambodia and Laos) and politically resistant (Myanmar)—attempted to increase state-led detection and reporting of outbreak events, significantly improving patterns of reporting. Of course, these improvements were not consistent or universal. There were differences among and within countries as well as among diseases. Yet the overall trend was clear and consistent, driven by a combination of peer pressure, an epistemic community of individuals in Ministries of Health, WHO regional offices, and the ASEAN secretariat, and political opportunities to progress transparent reporting behaviors. Diseases that were prioritized in the region and in funding programs, such as H5N1 and dengue, enjoyed more success when it came to generating reports than those that did not generate as much attention. The *political* obstacles to prompt and transparent reporting processes remained significant in several cases, as did problems of insufficient capacity to detect and report in a timely fashion in some countries, particularly Cambodia, Laos, and Myanmar. The system of detection and response in the Southeast Asian region proved both weak and strong in different situations: the strength of the system was its embeddedness in local capacity, local needs, and local politics—from this flowed the remarkable improvements in compliance. The weakness lay in the fact that prompt and open reporting rests on transparency and accountability within the broader political system, attributes that remain relatively rare in Southeast Asia. The impact of these problems in the wider political system on health performance is evident in how states in the region score on indexes like the Infectious Disease Vulnerability Index, where countries such as Cambodia, Laos, and Myanmar score as much "weaker" (twice as vulnerable) than their ASEAN neighbors (Moore et al. 2016).

Where progress has been achieved—in spite of political recalcitrance, commitment to sovereign noninterference, and capacity shortfalls—this has typically been due to donors and international actors, namely, the WHO, placing their trust in the capacity of existing regional institutions, namely, ASEAN, to cohere states around a persuasive argument that could be adapted to different political regimes, budgets, and health burdens. Regional ownership of APSED was vital. As I mentioned in chapter 2, most ASEAN states do not have abundant wealth reserves, a history of stability and prosperity, let alone a long-standing track record of social welfare and democratic governance. What was important for these states was the collective sense of shared fortune when it came to health emergencies. From lived experience, they learned that they depend on each other geographically and economically to survive outbreak events, to remain politically stable during outbreak events, and to build outbreak response capacity to ensure that endemic diseases are also being detected and managed. Living the consequence of this during Nipah, SARS, and then H5N1 meant that states were well primed to hear and respond to the constant refrain that the more state officials met each other to discuss APSED—the guidelines, the framework, the programs, the training, and the workshops—the better the cooperation and the greater the honest exchange among individual state participants on the obstacles they faced (Anonymous 2011a, 2011b, 2011c, 2012g, 2013b).

APSED—a new institution—played a pivotal role by serving as an inclusive network for combining political interests with technical knowledge as the region came to grips with the capacities required under the revised IHR. This unique regional model assisted in at least three crucial ways. First, by establishing an inclusive regional structure based on the cherished principles of noninterference and quiet diplomacy (namely, the avoidance of public criticism). Second, by facilitating the emergence of an epistemic community of experts linked by dense networks. Third, by maintaining the sense that the region confronted a common threat and had a shared regional purpose and responsibility to contain it. I will explore each of these in turn.

Regional Diplomacy

The first APSED phase established three regional dynamics critical to the implementation of the IHR. First, it moved beyond the structural separation of the WHO. APSED was a novel attempt to coordinate communication and engagement across two regions that were geographically linked but separated under the WHO management framework. This attempt, in and of itself, was a unique development for the WHO and regional partnership concerning disease outbreak response and detection. It points to the extent to which the impact of SARS and H5N1, followed by the adoption of the revised IHR, had entered the consciousness of all Asia Pacific states and led to a departure from politics as usual. APSED was designed to offer something to all members—from those ready to meet IHR core capacities to those a long way behind. Inclusion of diseases endemic to the region to test the applicability of the IHR core capacities was one local adaption provided to entice coordination and relevance across the membership. This inclusion was informal in practice, but, given the variety of states' capacity and health system strength, APSED was responsive in the first phase to the argument that IHR capacity building should be doing more than (just) assisting states with meeting IHR core capacities.

Second, APSED included political regional institutions such as ASEAN—to promote additional opportunities for partnership and dialogue among its SEARO and WPRO states. Crucially, the ASEAN secretariat was invited to the meetings organized around the five APSED programs, which led to coordination between APT EID Programme and the APSED phase. This created, for ASEAN states, a political and diplomatic commitment to APSED via ASEAN obligations. In Southeast Asia, state members were participating in APSED not only as individual WPRO or SEARO member states but also as ASEAN member states cognizant of their political and diplomatic commitments to ASEAN. Many technical and bureaucratic observers noted the difference this had on national-level discussions of APSED within ASEAN membership and the effect it had on potential political tensions that could have led to states abandoning the program or delivering little investment in the initiative.

Third, APSED tailored its approach, working methods, and priorities to suit regional needs and sensitivities, with a premium placed on building trust, recognizing regional interests, and respecting key principles (such as noninterference). Unity and trust were largely achieved by the avoidance of measurable targets on all 48 member states, and this left it vulnerable to critique. Those skeptical of the regional focus and who prefer a more global approach to IHR core capacity compliance pointed out the lack of measurable targets in the first phase of APSED. Those skeptical of the securitization lens adopted in the region to promote health system strengthening to meet the IHR core capacities stressed how APSED progressed a particular vision of IHR readiness that focused on detecting particular outbreaks, such as avian influenza, rather than building detection systems that could improve overall detection and readiness. The tension was that cooperation across the program areas required minimal political interference but maximum political support. How to unobtrusively measure an individual state's commitment to the principles of alert, response, and verification being promoted under APSED (as an expression of regional commitment to the revised IHR)? APSED enabled the tailoring of the IHR to regional circumstances in Southeast Asia. This created the possibility of implementation and behavioral change.

This approach was not, of course, without it downsides. Questions were raised about whether reliance on the "ASEAN way" norms helped conceal weak capacity and paper over the absence of political commitment in some cases. In 2011, when APSED entered its second phase, a shift emerged that reflected some of these concerns. Whereas Phase 1 of APSED had been careful to avoid individual state-based indicators, for fear of offending states or transgressing the principle of noninterference, Phase 2 (2010–2015) shifted to the adoption of a set of benchmarks for individual states to perform against. This was a deliberate attempt to demand more evidence from states, particularly in terms of matching their national plans to monitoring and evaluation (WPRO 2012). The IHR core capacities moved to center stage, and the regional adaption of the IHR was no longer a regional message but (literally) "for states to stake the recommendations and conclusions of these workshops seriously . . . for your governments to implement" (Anonymous 2011d). This was possible, politically, precisely because APSED Phase 1 had been so wary about singling out states and that, as a result, states had become increasingly comfortable with the process. Indeed, such was the level of comfort established that a SEARO official discussing Phase 2 noted with genuine concern that the bigger worry "this time" (in contrast to Phase 1) was not the lack of state commitment but donor fatigue. APSED had "translated the IHR into something that the region could understand," and his concern was that now avian influenza hadn't become the infectious disease it was feared; the budget infighting between WHO headquarters and the regional offices would lead to APSED becoming a program "versus" IHR programs at headquarters. The same official noted that, despite the regional specificity of APSED being its strength, "outsiders" (donors and WHO headquarters) were increasingly referring to it as a weakness (Anonymous 2010m).

Concern about the degree to which APSED permitted strong political relationships to flourish, possibly at the cost of technical improvements, was often raised at the sidelines of meetings. It was even hinted at in the evaluation of APSED's first phase report. However, APSED continued into Phase 2 with a focus on the five programs agreed to in Phase 1 and—again reflecting the region's stronger level of confidence—extended these to include three additional programs: public health emergency preparedness; regional preparedness, alert, and response; and, as discussed already, monitoring and evaluation (WPRO

2016: 13). In 2014, APSED's primary donors—Australia and the United States—proposed another independent evaluation of APSED to determine what had been achieved by Phase 2 and to provide recommendations on its future direction. The evaluation was performed in five member states (Indonesia, Laos, Mongolia, Nepal, and Viet Nam) (WPRO 2015: 54). It found that

> APSED has been useful to both regions. Member States' capabilities to detect, prepare for and respond to all public health events have been enhanced by the collective pursuit of a common goal using a common framework, proactive investment in capacities and a focus on generic capacities. (55)

Similar to the 2010 study, the 2014 evaluation found risk communication an ongoing problem for the region, with "mixed evidence of progress in the area of risk communication capacity, and many of the stakeholders consulted recognize that this is a challenging area, which requires greater emphasis on evaluating the effectiveness of communications." It recommended that "capacity-building will need to continue well beyond the final deadline for the achievement of IHR core capacities in 2016, and the end of APSED (2010)" (55). Overall, the 10-year anniversary evaluation of APSED found

> significant progress had been made. In particular, improvements were noted in the capacity of a number of Member States for surveillance, for human resource development through FETP, for laboratory capacity for diagnosis of priority and unknown diseases, and for communication between Member States and WHO through the IHR mechanism. However, the evaluation concluded all Member States in the Asia Pacific region remain vulnerable to emerging diseases and public health emergencies, and that challenges continued to exist in national and regional readiness to respond to large-scale and complex events in an effective and coordinated way. Multisectoral coordination remains challenging for Member States, however, the joint external evaluation (JEE) process for reviewing IHR implementation provides a means by which partners from different sectors collaborate and coordinate efforts to assess and provide recommendations on IHR implementation. The financial sustainability of core public health programmes also remains challenging. (WPRO 2016: 14)

The report noted that while significant challenges remained—not least, vulnerability to disease, multisectoral coordination, and financial sustainability—significant progress continued to be made. In other words, despite all the challenges, states were continuing to cooperate to implement their commitments to the IHR.

Key to this sustained progress, I argue, is the politics underlying it—the regional diplomacy facilitated by APSED, which helps set shared regional expectations (irrespective of political regimes) and facilitates problem solving in political sensitive ways. One concern for the future is that the politics may become undervalued and technical capacity given preference. This was a risk in the second phase, as the program moved to emphasize individual states' obligation—over the collective obligation—to fulfill APSED programs. In practice, the shift from a focus on the political to a focus on the technical can be seen in the shift from prioritizing regional cooperation to a focus on national technical capabilities. This was evident during Phase 2, when donors placed the emphasis squarely on the idea that regional resilience in an outbreak emergency depends upon the strength of national response. Although regional cooperation appears still to be the mechanism through which APSED is promoted and delivered, particularly apparent is the diminishing role of APT, which was so crucial at the outset.

As noted in the recent Australian government study on its decade of investment in regional health security, while APSED has been important for communicating technical support and technical expertise in the region, ASEAN's and APT's roles have become somewhat neglected (Australian Government 2017: 127). This is evidenced in the fact that ASEAN statements and APT-related statements on emerging infectious disease and communicable disease become rarer after 2010, as did the funding. Yet APT was vital in developing an additional dedicated space for SEARO and WPRO states to discuss APSED, which served to reinforce the political message of IHR compliance. The problem for donors is that these awareness-raising activities are difficult to evaluate and measure, and outbreak events like Ebola overtake the (longer-term) investments in political cooperation in preference for short-term, easily measured investments in technical capacity. Equally, APSED's success was a problem for WHO headquarters' attempt to assert its international governance role (and save its diminishing budget).

As such, external actors' (donor states and WHO headquarters) fixation on technical capacity and investment in national performance to meet the IHR core capacities was already strong in the second APSED phase, and it intensified after the Ebola outbreak in West Africa. A view repeatedly iterated after the Ebola outbreak was that the annual IHR capacity self-reporting structure was too generic, and it has permitted many states to avoid serious questions about their performance (Gostin et al. 2016). It was argued that recalcitrant states could sit in groups like AFRO, EMRO, SEARO, WPRO, and PAHO—even a more IHR-focused program like APSED—without being called out for their individual shortfalls across the eight IHR core capacities. Moreover, in a post-2009 global financial crisis era, donor states were no longer keen to fund initiatives that did not demonstrate measurable improvements of performance (Sridhar, Winters, and Strong 2017). While the APSED 10-year anniversary report acknowledged the importance of APSED as a regional forum that maintains momentum and focus on collective containment strategy and program building, there was also a clear message that individual states were "getting away" with hiding their capacity shortfall among the crowd (WPRO 2015).

In this context, the recent WHO JEE initiative has emerged as the principal means of targeting investment and monitoring at individual state pandemic preparedness in the post-Ebola era. The JEE was originally led by the Global Health Security Agenda, which was formed as a multilateral steering group of 10 countries: Canada, Chile, Finland, India, Indonesia, Italy, Kenya, the Kingdom of Saudi Arabia, the Republic of Korea, and the United States. The GHSA, headquartered in South Korea, where the initiative was launched in February 2014, is very much a US-funded initiative that finances "action packages" for states that agree to "focus their efforts on achieving specific targets. All GHSA countries have flexibility in how they address their commitments, with countries working nationally, regionally, and/or globally toward the common targets" (GHSA 2016). In the first five-year phase $1 billion was invested in 17 countries (called Phase 1 countries). From within the WPRO and SEARO, five countries were identified for investment: Bangladesh, Indonesia, India, Pakistan, and, from Southeast Asia, Viet Nam. Phase 2 countries (14 in total) were also identified as having an opportunity to develop programs and targets with GHSA. From the Asian region these included Cambodia, Laos, Malaysia, and Thailand. It is not clear what selection criteria was used to identify which states went into which phase; funding, training, and workshops began in 2015, and other donors were invited to contribute (G7 countries, G20 countries, Nordic countries, Australia, and international organizations were included in all the events) (3–4).

There are eleven action packages that countries may select to dedicate their action toward: Prevent 1: Antimicrobial Resistance; Prevent 2: Zoonotic Disease; Prevent 3: Biosafety and Biosecurity; Prevent 4: Immunization; Detect 1: National Laboratory System; Detect 2 and Detect 3: Real-Time Surveillance; Detect 4: Reporting; Detect 5: Workforce Development; Respond 1: Emergency Operations Centres; Respond 2: Linking Public Health with Law and Multisectoral Rapid Response; Respond 3: Medical Countermeasures and Personnel

Deployment. Emphasis is squarely on states identifying their own action focus, developing a road map to achieve action, and dedicating local resources to achieve this focus. Assessments occur at two stages: country self-assessment and then external assessment—the JEE, which includes IHR core capacity measures that a state's action and performance are measured against. After Ebola, the JEE GHSA assessment became aligned with the WHO headquarters Joint Evaluation Exercise assessment. This JEE was introduced in 2015 on the recommendation of the IHR Review Committee on Second Extensions for Establishing National Public Health Capacities and on IHR Implementation (WHA 2016a).

The JEE arose out of concerns, stemming from the Ebola outbreak, that self-assessment of IHR core capacities was permitting states to avoid critical self-evaluation of capacity. What is more, Western (donor) governments and the WHO were concerned that, globally, the political momentum to change in line with IHR compliance was becoming exhausted (WHO 2016b: 1–2). The Australian and Finnish governments therefore created an alliance—the JEE Alliance—to encourage countries to participate in dialogue and exchanges on the baseline targets for IHR compliance to be JEE ready. Countries may individually opt in to all these schemes—the GHSA and the JEE Alliance—on the assumption that those that do can leverage participation for additional external investment. The logic is that the political and financial rewards from opting in will have a snowball effect to the point where those who do not opt in are perceived as having something to hide, as not being cooperative regional members in the project of health security, and maybe not the safest destinations for travel and trade (although these points are never made in the promotional material).

The steering committee of the GHSA is a deliberate hybrid of states are different income levels, and the UK and the United States put themselves forward for the first JEE GHSA assessments in 2015. In the JEE Alliance, created in 2016, which has a platform of 64 members including countries and non-state actors (including the WHO, the World Bank, and the Bill and Melinda Gates Foundation), emphasis is on common challenges that actors meet together to address health security: "transparency in exchanging information, supports linking national planning and implementation to follow on the results of evaluations, and aims at creating innovative solutions and opportunities for supporting country capacity building" (JEE Alliance 2017). The country membership of the JEE Alliance from the Asian region includes Bangladesh, Cambodia, Indonesia,

Nepal, Pakistan, and the Republic of Korea. The JEE is a voluntary process that a country requests from the WHO to conduct an external evaluation of its public health emergency preparedness and to progress toward IHR core capacities. In the SEARO and WPRO regions, nine countries to date have requested an evaluation: Bangladesh, Cambodia, Laos, the Maldives, Mongolia, Myanmar, Sri Lanka, Thailand, and Viet Nam.

This all appears to be moving health security in the right direction—a focus on individual capacity and supporting incremental actions to achieve the eight IHR core capacities. Yet although these new initiatives go out of their way to be nonhegemonic, both have a distinct North-South character inconsistent with the regional approach adopted by Southeast Asia in APSED Phase 1. As a result, these programs risk losing regional ownership. Southeast Asian states may individually choose to opt in, or out, but their capacity to drive and lead the initiative is heavily curtailed. Nor are these schemes consistent with regional norms, drawing instead from Western diplomatic practices, including naming and shaming. This carries risks that individual governments may become alienated and a longer-term danger that the regional peer pressure, epistemic engagement, and political persuasion that came from the earlier regional engagement will become weaker going forward. The sense of common threat, the dense networks among neighboring states, and the normative pull of regional security was the glue that held APSED Phase 1 together and propelled states to understand that IHR compliance was a collective, not individual, endeavor. Although new programs are meritorious in their own right, they could unintentionally weaken the existing foundations of regional cooperation.

Dense Networks

The 2015 APSED report noted that Southeast Asia had become increasingly comfortable with reporting outbreak events. This was exemplified by the creation of two new regional journals, the *Western Pacific Surveillance and Response Journal* (*WPSAR*) and the *WHO South East Asia Journal of Public Health* (*WPSAR*'s first volume was published in 2010, and *South East Asia Journal* followed in 2012), designed in part for that purpose. Outbreaks were not to be treated as shameful events illustrative of weak health systems. Instead, outbreak events became research opportunities with honest, reflective pieces that included ministry-led or ministry-coauthored analysis of an outbreak, the response, the effectiveness of the plan to contain, and the all-important lessons learned. This has resulted in the normalization of shared outbreak communication—as the APSED 2015 report noted (WPRO 2015: 46): between 2014 and 2015 alone eight articles were published in *WPSAR* on outbreak events from within the region.

The creation of open-access journals illustrates how effective APSED and its first-phase champions were in promoting a regional culture of research, exchange, and trust in the area of outbreak response. As the first paper published in the journal by WPRO epidemiologist and editor Emma Field and then-director of the WPRO Communicable Disease Unit Takeshi Kasai said:

> Further evidence highlighting the need for a publication for the Western Pacific Region was demonstrated during the 2009 pandemic when authors in the Western Pacific Region published surveillance reports in the European-focused journal, *Eurosurveillance*. (Field and Kasai 2010: 1)

This illustrates an important but overlooked aspect of APSED Phase 1—it was a local adaption of an international instrument. That was the point. Situating IHR compliance within regional experience and a regional network was vital. It was a "shared normative understanding of regional order" (Acharya 2009: 148) that promoted regional cooperation among ASEAN states because it approached its task in a manner consistent with existing norms and practices (Foot 2014: 199–200). The novelty of APSED was that it further encouraged states to understand that their security was tied fundamentally to a regional enterprise—that, in other words, their own fate was tied to that of others. APSED created a regional network that spanned two WHO regional offices and multiple regional institutions, financial institutions, and bilateral arrangements. It was inclusive, with membership granted irrespective of regime type or health system capacity. Until then, states with weak health system capacity had used that weakness as an excuse to justify noncompliance with their obligation to detect and report. Meanwhile, states used to concealing information from their citizens were for the first time put under significant peer pressure to rethink whether secrecy made them more or less secure, nudging them toward stronger compliance. This is precisely why states such as Viet Nam attempted to improve their reporting behavior and why those such as Cambodia and Laos speak honestly in APSED program forums about the material challenges they confronted. The establishment of regional networks of experts helped created peer pressure that strongly encouraged greater compliance. Even Myanmar started to improve its reporting behavior, albeit marginally, during Phase 1 (see chap. 5). Such shifts were the product of political calculations taken after exposure to a regional network that normalized cooperation and communication.

Common Threat

I noted above that a "shared normative understanding of regional order" (Acharya 2009: 148) created moments of genuine cooperation among ASEAN states. We need to take notice of when and where ASEAN states began to conceptualize their own interests and prosperity as being tied to the fate of the region more broadly and achieved through collective action, since this was crucial in re-shaping behavior. What ASEAN states learned through painful experience with infectious disease outbreaks was that the principal threat was not just the fact of an outbreak but of a neighboring state being incapable of containing an outbreak, and the region, in turn, being unable to contain the spread. Therefore, the referent object being secured in APSED was not individual patients, or groups, or health professionals—it was the state itself, but the nature of the threat it confronted was necessarily transnational and thus required a transnational response. The purpose of APSED was carefully crafted—to assist states with reconceptualizing the function of a responsible sovereign in the post-SARS world. A responsible sovereign capable of containment—and therefore free from interference—fits the self-identity of most ASEAN states. As I showed in chapters 2 and 3, most ASEAN states have pursued health systems strengthening as well as health security with zeal after their individual emergence from conflict (Myanmar remains the exception). APSED bound states together, particularly ASEAN states, because of this shared understanding of the common threat. The threat was demonstrated by SARS and then solidified in the minds of the region's political leaders by H5N1. Cooperation would be the only way to survive but what system of reform could accommodate such different political regimes and capacities? As chapter 4 discussed, APSED went a long way to provide this answer. Spanning subregions, emerging threats like H5N1, and endemic ones like dengue, this program sought out technical expertise and political engagement as a mutually constitutive endeavor. ASEAN states, in particular, responded positively to this program because it did not threaten the core purpose of ASEAN unity—its actually strengthened the capability and function of the sovereign state.

The limits of this approach, as I identified in chapters 5 and 6, becomes acute when the state refuses to make the necessary reforms or dedicate sufficient resources to the task. When states fail to fulfill their responsibility, mistrust is bred within society. At the same time, overly statist approaches can take agency away from individuals and non-state actors. This can reduce the overall capacity committed to risk communication messages and supporting the state in detecting and verifying outbreaks and deal with the effects. States may dissuade community and provincial health workers from reporting honestly, health care workers may independently decide not to report in order to protect communities or avoid repercussions for communicating outside the political chain of command. There are a number of states within ASEAN—in particular, Cambodia, Myanmar, and Laos—in which health workers have had to make these decisions.

APSED, in its first phase, came closest to having these discussions about the common threat, which was not the outbreak per se but states' incapacity to mount an effective and transparent response to an outbreak. However, as a result of the Ebola crisis in 2014 and increasing need for monitoring and evaluation criteria in aid packages, there has been a shift away from the communicative, relational, and facilitative purposes of APSED—its conversations and rituals—toward a much narrower focus on individual state compliance with the IHR core capacities. Under programs like the JEE Alliance, the risk is that the conversation shifts from regional functions and cooperation to individual state function. One engagement must not replace the other. Emphasis on individual state IHR compliance could obscure the regional level as an (opportunistic) site for dialogue, technical support, and peer pressure. Without that, ownership and peer pressure are diminished, and implementation becomes less sensitive to regional norms. In that context, it becomes gradually easier for states to avoid compliance and revert to noninterference behavior. In a region such as ASEAN, this is illustrated in the fact that having laboratories and legislation prepared for an emergency also requires states to adapt their political function to accommodate open sources of communication, familiarize health and bureaucratic staff with communicating outbreak situations, and normalizing cooperative operations so that the system—and populations—are ready to trust and support government responses in an emergency.

In APSED's first phase the common threat narrative was refined and tailored to regional experiences and concerns. This enabled ownership and commitment. States could not deny their responsibility to try to improve detection, reporting, and communication because they were the architects of the program. Ownership and empowerment in disease outbreak response remains vital to achieve state-level engagement with the function of being a prepared state.

To Protect Health, Secure the Politics

The 2007 WHO *World Health Report* concluded that professionals and policy makers in the fields of public health, foreign policy, and national security should maintain open dialogue on endemic diseases and practices that pose personal health threats, including HIV/AIDS, which also have the potential to threaten national and international health security. The states that could talk openly about their capacity to respond to endemic and epidemic diseases would be the ones most secure when facing the next outbreak. In Southeast Asia, what may have started as rhetoric about health security became the foundational elements that pulled together a regional network that compelled states to think *regionally* when deciding how to detect, report, and communicate disease outbreak events (Australian Government 2017: 117). The region is a crucial intersection between the concrete domestic context and the abstract international environment.

The regional adaption of the revised IHR embodied in APSED served as a crucial foundation on which the region was able to explore the demands of the revised IHR. APSED provided a guide to prioritize and adapt capacities to the region's needs. The regional model assisted in the three crucial ways. First, it allowed states to discuss the challenges they faced and identify the assistance they needed in a context sensitive to regional norms, interests, and values. Second, the tripartite model, which included ASEAN, the WPRO, and SEARO under APSED, overcame regional divisions by permitting states of different economies, politics, and capacities to sit in the same room to discuss their regional health threats. Third, the identification of a shared regional threat established a common element necessary for action: a shared interest. From that sprang a sense of common regional responsibility to contain it, irrespective of capacity. However, capacity shortfalls and disagreements remained. Indeed, these shortfalls remain a concern for ASEAN and should be considered in any discussion of lessons learned from APSED. Identification of a shared threat and a shared responsibility does not generate sufficient shared capacity by itself (Wenham 2016). There were tensions in how APSED prioritized, ultimately, infectious disease outbreak containment, given serious health system financial and disease burdens in countries in the region that have not yet met their IHR core capacity requirements. Comfort with reporting outbreak events has improved but here too, behind the underlying trends, sit significant differences of performance. Verifying an outbreak is as important as detecting the outbreak if it is to be contained. Having the diagnostic capacity to verify an outbreak remains an outstanding concern for a number of ASEAN countries. Asking a neighboring state for assistance with diagnostics does not appear to have become embedded practice yet, and as a result there have been instances of tension between states with disease outbreaks reaching their borders without prior notice.

Regional health security became the conduit through which states sought to encourage their neighbors to become responsive to some of the political aspects of containing a disease outbreak—including the need for transparent and prompt communication. The great strength of the approach taken in Southeast Asia was its political dimension, its sensitivity to regional norms and interests, and the buy-in of regional institutions. It was precisely this sensitivity and buy-in that facilitated the improved reporting performance I identified earlier. But, by the end of APSED Phase 2 in 2015, this political dimension diminished in donor preference for states to attach themselves to individual evaluations, exercises, and training in schemes like GHSA and JEE—agendas largely driven by actors primarily outside the region. These individual capacity-building mechanisms are important, but they should not replace regional processes that encourage states to communicate their understanding of shared expectations, facilitate regional ownership, and exhibit consistency with regional norms and values.

Immediately after the Ebola outbreak in West Africa, WHO headquarters looked to deflect criticism of its performance by attributing the failed response almost entirely to dysfunction and mismanagement in the African regional office. Whatever the merits of this line of argument—and there was no escaping the fact that Geneva must accept a significant share of the blame—this led to important changes to the disease reporting process, which now requires that states communicate a suspected directly outbreak to WHO headquarters (and not to WHO regional offices, as had continued to occur after the IHR revisions in 2005). The image of an organization held hostage to its decentralized Cold War structure, in drastic need of reform, was powerful. Of course, this image does not convey the rivalry and competition within the WHO, especially the desire for locating political power at headquarters.

To be sure, there are vast differences within and among the WHO regional offices. APSED revealed the differences and the tension—the WPRO is by all accounts well financed and organized, while SEARO remains less well financed and struggles to be responsive to individual state requests for assistance. When each regional office took turns in managing APSED from year to year, in the first phase, there was much frustration expressed by the WPRO that the program was better managed when it was in charge. However, there was also a feeling that increasingly united the WPRO and SEARO—the original support from WHO headquarters for a biregional strategy to build IHR compliance. The concern is whether this support has given way to a new sentiment in WHO headquarters—that the IHR and their functions not remain a function of regional offices. Headquarters support for APSED diminished as the years rolled by. The role of APSED in IHR implementation discussions was increasingly minimized even among WHO headquarters staff. This shift in attitude was one that the author witnessed. Full-throated support from Geneva for a regional approach to implementation had given way by 2015. Interviews with WHO headquarters in 2008 produced a very different response to questions about APSED in 2015: "APSED is dead. It is irrelevant" (Anonymous 2015b).

Now in the third phase of APSED (2015–2020), we should not forget what its first phase achieved. Nor should we diminish the odds that were stacked against this initiative. Southeast Asia, a region committed to noninterference and sovereignty, opened up to the idea of collective disease reporting and surveillance behavior. These states especially put that idea into practice in the form of improved reporting performance within the region. The revised IHR ambition of prompt and proactive detection was progressed through the engagement of regional institutions, the establishment of formal and informal mechanisms that responded to local sensitivities and shared regional norms, and the generation of epistemic communities. These were forged out of a regional understanding of shared threat and common destiny that was discussed not in the halls of Geneva but in shared lived experience and fear of infectious disease in the region. For Southeast Asia's improved performance in the detection and reporting of infectious disease to be maintained and progressed into the future, it will be imperative that the region's own politics, norms, state institutions, and civil society remain at the forefront in shaping the direction and implementation of policies for health security.

IHR Core Capacity Compliance Data 2010 and 2015

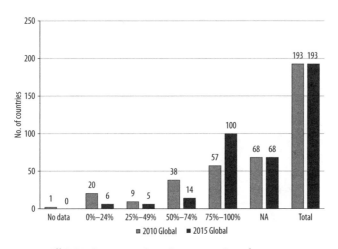

Figure A.1. All IHR Countries Core Capacity 1: Legislation, 2010 vs. 2015

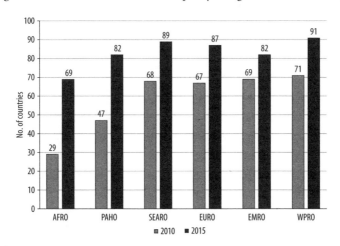

Figure A.2. WHO States Implementation of Legislation, 2010 vs. 2015

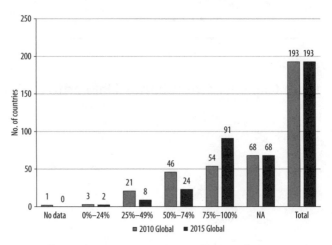

Figure A.3. All IHR Countries Core Capacity 2: Coordination, 2010 vs. 2015

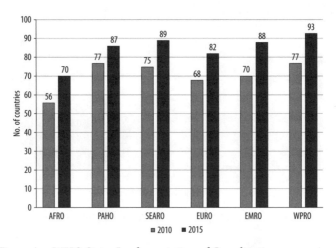

Figure A.4. WHO States Implementation of Coordination, 2010 vs. 2015

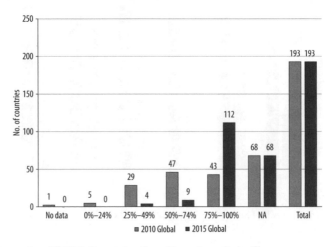

Figure A.5. All IHR Countries Core Capacity 3: Surveillance, 2010 vs. 2015

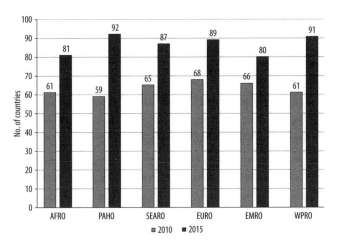

Figure A.6. WHO States Implementation of Surveillance, 2010 vs. 2015

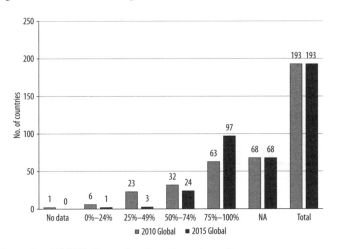

Figure A.7. All IHR Countries Core Capacity 4: Response, 2010 vs. 2015

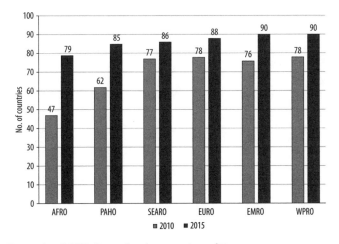

Figure A.8. WHO States Implementation of Response, 2010 vs. 2015

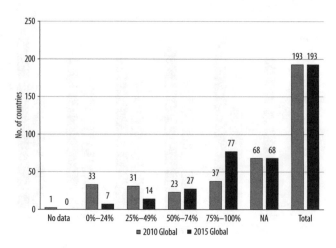

Figure A.9. All IHR Countries Core Capacity 5: Preparedness, 2010 vs. 2015

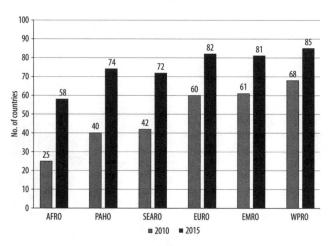

Figure A.10. WHO States Implementation of Preparedness, 2010 vs. 2015

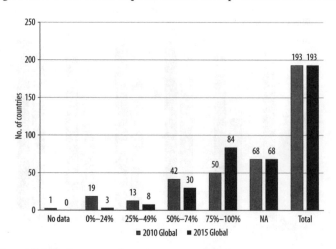

Figure A.11. All IHR Countries Core Capacity 6: Risk Communication, 2010 vs. 2015

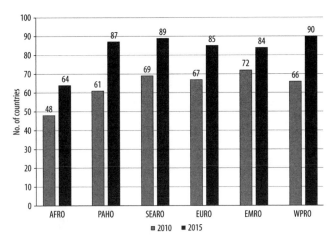

Figure A.12. WHO States Implementation of Risk Communication, 2010 vs. 2015

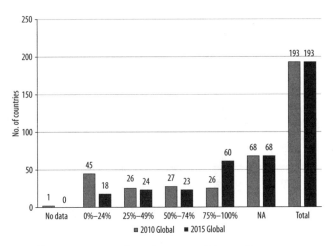

Figure A.13. All IHR Countries Core Capacity 7: Human Resources, 2010 vs. 2015

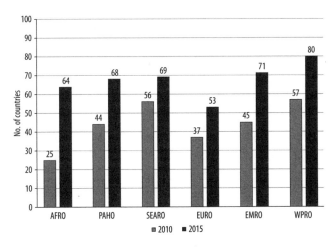

Figure A.14. WHO States Implementation of Human Resources, 2010 vs. 2015

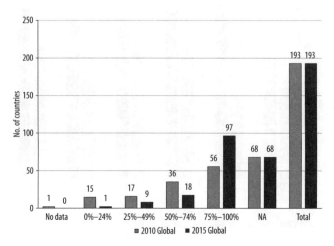

Figure A.15. All IHR Countries Core Capacity 8: Laboratory, 2010 vs. 2015

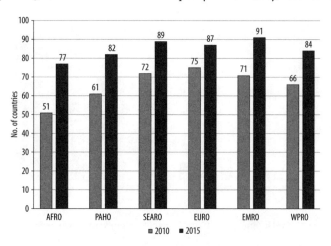

Figure A.16. WHO States Implementation of Laboratory, 2010 vs. 2015

Introduction

1. A PHEIC is defined in the revised IHR as "an extraordinary event [irrespective of origin or source] which: (i) constitutes a public health risk to other States through the international spread of disease and (ii) potentially require(s) a coordinated international response" (WHA 2005: 8).

2. ASEAN member states under SEARO governance are Indonesia, Myanmar, and Thailand.

3. ASEAN member states under WPRO governance are Brunei Darussalam, Cambodia, China (People's Republic of), Lao (People's Democratic Republic), Malaysia, Philippines, Singapore, and Viet Nam.

4. Detecting and reporting infectious diseases enable the other capacities to follow, as has been noted in general regarding the majority of states that have met some but not all of the IHR core capacity requirements (Ijaz et al. 2012: 1054–1057).

5. Similar arguments have been put forward promoting looser regional formations to facilitate IHR compliance sometimes through formal regional organizations (but sometimes not); see Gresham et al. 2013; Kasolo et al. 2013.

6. Gostin and Katz (2016) identify from the eight reviews conducted between 2014 and 2016 at least 10 recommendations and suggest 11 of their own.

Chapter 1 · The Revised International Health Regulations in Practice

1. The two original goals of the IHR: limit the spread of disease and reduce interference with the flow of travel and trade.

2. The year the WHO was created and was assigned responsibility for the International Sanitary Convention.

3. The WHO Constitution ([1948] 2009) details:

Article 21
The Health Assembly shall have authority to adopt regulations concerning:
(a) sanitary and quarantine requirements and other procedures designed to prevent the international spread of disease;
(b) nomenclatures with respect to diseases, causes of death and public health practices;
(c) standards with respect to diagnostic procedures for international use;
(d) standards with respect to the safety, purity and potency of biological, pharmaceutical and similar products moving in international commerce;
(e) advertising and labelling of biological, pharmaceutical and similar products moving in international commerce.

Article 22
Regulations adopted pursuant to Article 21 shall come into force for all Members after due notice has been given of their adoption by the Health Assembly except for such

Members as may notify the Director-General of rejection or reservations within the period stated in the notice.

4. This was not to be the case. The first convention to appear before the WHA and be adopted was the Framework Convention on Tobacco Control in 2003 (Wipfli 2015).

5. Because the IHR remain a regulation (not a convention) it has the signature of all member states of the WHA unless reservations to particular articles or the instrument itself are submitted to the WHA.

6. For a detailed account of the events that transpired during the Ebola outbreak in West Africa, see the collection of chapters and vignettes in Hofman and Au 2017.

7. It is important to note there are those who challenge this view; see McInnes 2015; and Kamradt-Scott 2016.

8. The source used for this section is the International Health Regulations (2005) Monitoring Framework, WHO Global Health Observatory (GHO) data repository. www.who.int/gho/ihr/en/.

9. Across the five regions, the most heavily indebted poor countries are in the African region (30 countries out of 36 listed heavily indebted poor countries) (World Bank 2016: 1).

10. See the appendix for graphs of each IHR core capacity, comparing 2010 reported data with 2015 reported data. The breakdown of data is by WHO region and informs the discussion on pp. 36–38.

Chapter 2 · The Political Context in Southeast Asia

1. This is emerging; see Ottersen et al. 2014.

2. Of additional benefit, measures exist on infectious disease prevalence for the period of study (particularly HIV, malaria, TB), maternal mortality data (the indicators most often referenced by both health insecurity and democracy studies), and defense and public health expenditure for the region.

3. Perlo-Freeman uses simple regression to look at the relationship among welfare expenditure, military expenditure, and health-education outcomes; however, that study does not examine the effect of postconflict recovery and regime type.

4. Defined by the membership of ASEAN, which includes Brunei, Cambodia, Indonesia, Laos, Malaysia, Myanmar, Philippines, Singapore, Thailand, and Viet Nam.

5. The TB DALY measure for Viet Nam had dramatically improved by 2010.

Chapter 3 · Sovereignty, Regional Cooperation, and Health Security

1. (1) Early-warning surveillance and response, (2) laboratory strengthening, (3) infection control, (4) risk communication, and (5) enhanced regional and international collaboration.

2. Cambodia, Laos, Indonesia, Malaysia (suspect poultry cases in 2005 and 2006), Myanmar (suspect poultry and human cases in 2006 and 2007), the Philippines (suspect poultry cases in 2006 and 2007), Thailand, and Viet Nam.

3. American Samoa; Australia; Brunei Darussalam; Cambodia; China; the Cook Islands; Fiji; French Polynesia (France); Guam (USA); Hong Kong (China); Japan; Kiribati; the Lao People's Democratic Republic; Macao (China); Malaysia; the Marshall Islands; Micronesia, Federated States of; Mongolia; Nauru; New Caledonia (France); New Zealand; Niue; Northern Mariana Islands, Commonwealth of the; Palau; Papua New Guinea; the Philippines; the Pitcairn Islands (UK); the Republic of Korea; Samoa; Singapore; the Solomon Islands; Tokelau (associate member, New Zealand); Tonga; Tuvalu; Vanuatu; Viet Nam; Wallis and Futuna.

4. The first H5N1 outbreak case was in 1997 in Hong Kong.

Chapter 4 · Forging Political Support

1. Indonesia remains the worst-affected country in the world with H5N1 cases.

2. The first H5N1 outbreak case was in 1997 in Hong Kong, but it remained on the island.

3. SEARO membership consists of Bangladesh, Bhutan, the Democratic Republic of Korea, India, Indonesia, the Maldives, Myanmar, Nepal, Sri Lanka, Thailand, and Timor Leste.

WPRO membership consists of American Samoa (USA), New Caledonia (France), Australia, New Zealand, Brunei Darussalam, Niue, Cambodia, the Commonwealth of the Northern Mariana Islands (USA), China, Palau, the Cook Islands, Papua New Guinea, Fiji, the Philippines, French Polynesia (France), the Pitcairn Islands (UK), Guam (USA), the Republic of Korea, Hong Kong (China), Samoa, Japan, Singapore, Kiribati, the Solomon Islands, Lao People's Democratic Republic, Tokelau (New Zealand), Macao (China), Tonga, Malaysia, Tuvalu, the Marshall Islands, Vanuatu, the Federated States of Micronesia, Viet Nam, Mongolia, Wallis and Futuna (France), and Nauru.

4. In 2008–2009, SEARO had an annual budget of US$363 million (with US$103 million accessed contributions, the remainder voluntary contributions); while WPRO in same year had a US$230 million total, with US$79 million from accessed contributions (WPR/RC61/4 2010: 14).

5. China did provide a declaration in May 2007 pertaining to how its federal health structure would meet the IHR core capacity requirements; India presented a reservation on 14 December 2006—but one that sought to expand the IHR revisions to include yellow fever for the Indian state. See http://www.who.int/ihr/legal_issues/states_parties/en/index.html.

6. "On the record" and "off the record" TAG (hardcopy) transcripts from 2006 to 2010 are held by the author.

7. See http://apps.who.int/iris/bitstream/handle/10665/126793/rdr60_CDS.pdf?sequence =7, p. 6; http://apps.who.int/iris/bitstream/handle/10665/206349/B1391.pdf?sequence=1&ua=1, pp. 15–16, 27.

8. Though the acronym APSED includes "Asia Pacific," the APSED review in 2010 reported a widely understood failure to incorporate the Pacific into its five program areas, and this became a key focus for the second APSED phase (2010–2015) (Heywood and Moussavi 2010: 36).

Chapter 5 · Surveillance and Reporting in Practice

1. Brunei Darussalam is a member of ASEAN and the WPRO, but there are no data presented for Brunei in the tables. Not one report was provided by Brunei or on Brunei for the duration of the period examined, 1996–2010. Brunei Darussalam is a small country of just under 500,000 people; however, it did attend all the APSED and APT EID functions held concerning IHR compliance and readiness. Brunei also provided a self-report survey on its IHR core capacity performance in 2010.

2. The PMM has since joined analytical forces with HealthMap and now has a text-mining algorithm capability (search all news media source providers in multiple languages for outbreak reports).

3. Public health assessment under the IHR requires states to determine whether an outbreak should be notified to the international community according to four criteria:

1. Is the public health impact of the event serious? (yes/no)
2. Is the event unusual or unexpected? (yes/no)
3. Is there any significant risk of international spread? (yes/no)
4. Is there any significant risk of international travel or trade restrictions? (yes/no) (WHO/ HSE/IHR/2010.4: 14)

4. But there is little evidence of incident reporting on the SEARO site in spite of its large outbreak cases per year. See Heffelfinger et al. 2017.

Chapter 6 · Understanding the Differences in Reporting Responsibilities

1. For example, there is no reference to human rights response in the one-year review by the WHO nor in the independent review; see WHA 2016a; 2016b. In fact, it has been noted that the WHO appears determined to focus on a narrative that is only positive about its role in the Ebola outbreak; see Oxfam International 2015: 4.

2. It should be noted that 2012 was the first cutoff date for 100% core capacity compliance.

Primary Sources

Interviews (transcripts held with author)

Anonymous. 2007a. WHO official. November. Geneva, Switzerland.

Anonymous. 2007b. WHO official. November. Geneva, Switzerland.

Anonymous. 2007c. WHO official. November. Geneva, Switzerland.

Anonymous 2008a. International Division official. Department of Health and Aging. April. Canberra, Australia.

Anonymous. 2008b. ASEAN official. June. Melbourne, Australia.

Anonymous. 2008c. WPRO official. September. Manila, Philippines.

Anonymous. 2008d. WPRO official. September. Manila, Philippines.

Anonymous. 2008e. Health Ministry official. September. Manila, Philippines.

Anonymous. 2008f. Department of Foreign Affairs and Trade official. November. Canberra, Australia.

Anonymous. 2010a. APSED TAG member. May. Brisbane, Australia.

Anonymous. 2010b. Health Ministry official. October. Hanoi, Viet Nam.

Anonymous. 2010c. Health Ministry official. October. Hanoi, Viet Nam.

Anonymous. 2010d. World Bank official. October. Hanoi, Viet Nam.

Anonymous. 2010e. WHO official. October. Hanoi, Viet Nam.

Anonymous. 2010f. UNDP official. October, Hanoi, Viet Nam.

Anonymous. 2010g. Health Ministry official. October. Phnom Penh, Cambodia.

Anonymous. 2010h. WHO official. October. Phnom Penh, Cambodia.

Anonymous. 2010i. NGO official. October. Phnom Penh, Cambodia.

Anonymous. 2010j. Health Ministry official. October. Jakarta, Indonesia.

Anonymous. 2010k. Health Ministry official. October. Jakarta, Indonesia.

Anonymous. 2010l. WHO official. October. Jakarta, Indonesia.

Anonymous. 2010m. SEARO official. October. Jakarta, Indonesia.

Anonymous. 2010n. GPHIN official (Canada). November. Phone interview.

Anonymous. 2010o. Health Division. AusAID official. November. Canberra, Australia.

Anonymous. 2010p. APSED Evaluation Team. AusAID official. November. Canberra, Australia.

Anonymous. 2010q. APSED Evaluation Team. AusAID official. November. Canberra, Australia.

Anonymous. 2011a. Health Ministry official (Laos). November. Manila, Philippines.

Anonymous. 2011b. Health Ministry official (Myanmar). November. Manila, Philippines.

Anonymous. 2011c. ASEAN official. November. Manila, Philippines.

Anonymous. 2011d. Former WHO HQ official. November. Manila, Philippines.

Anonymous. 2011e. SEARO official. November. Manila, Philippines.

Anonymous. 2012a. ASEAN official. July. Interview. Follow-up e-mail. Brisbane, Australia.

Anonymous. 2012b. SEARO official. September. Phone interview. Follow-up e-mail.

Anonymous. 2012c. Mekong Basin Disease Surveillance official. October. Bangkok, Thailand.

Anonymous. 2012d. Health Ministry official. October. Bangkok, Thailand.

Anonymous. 2012e. Health Ministry official. October. Bangkok, Thailand.
Anonymous. 2012f. Health Ministry official. October. Putrajaya, Malaysia.
Anonymous. 2012g. Health Ministry focus group interview. October. Putrajaya, Malaysia.
Anonymous. 2013a. ASEAN official (former). April. Bali, Indonesia.
Anonymous. 2013b. Health Ministry official (New Zealand). April. Bali, Indonesia.
Anonymous. 2014. GPHIN official (Canada). February. Ottawa, Canada.
Anonymous. 2015a. ProMED official. December. London, United Kingdom.
Anonymous. 2015b. WHO official. December. London, United Kingdom.

Primary Documents (copies held with author)

ProMED-mail. Search Archive. www.promedmail.org.
Western Pacific Regional Office (WPRO). 2012. Informal Consultation on Public Health Emergency Planning. 15–16 March, Manila, Philippines. Files held with author.
Western Pacific Regional Office (WPRO). 2011. Workshop on Risk Communication for Public Health Emergencies, 15–17 November, Manila, Philippines. Files held with author.
Western Pacific Regional Office and South-East Asia Regional Office (WPRO-SEARO). 2005–2013. Reports of the Asia Pacific Technical Advisory Group (TAG) and bi-regional meeting for APSED, Phase 1 and Phase 2. Files held with author.
WHO for the Western Pacific Regional Office (WPRO). Documents and provisional summary records (SEARCH: emerging infectious disease(s), infectious disease(s), surveillance, International Health Regulations, APSED, ASEAN), World Health Organization Regional Committee for the Western Pacific, Fifty-Sixth Session (2005), Fifty-Seventh Session (2006), Fifty-Eighth Session (2007), Fifty-Ninth Session (2008), Sixtieth Session (2009), Sixty-First Session (2010), Sixty-Second Session (2011), Sixty-Third Session (2012). Files held with author.
WHO South-East Asia Regional Office (SEARO). Documents and provisional summary records (SEARCH: emerging infectious disease(s), infectious disease(s), surveillance, International Health Regulations, APSED, ASEAN), World Health Organization Regional Committee for South-East Asia, Fifty-Sixth Session (2005), Fifty-Seventh Session (2006), Fifty-Eighth Session (2007), Fifty-Ninth Session (2008), Sixtieth Session (2009), Sixty-First Session (2010), Sixty-Second Session (2011), Sixty-Third Session (2012). Files held with author.
World Health Organization (WHO). *Disease Outbreak News* (*DON*). 1996–2017. www.who.int/csr/don/en/.
World Health Organization (WHO). Documents and provisional summary records (SEARCH: emerging infectious disease(s), infectious disease(s), surveillance, International Health Regulations, APSED, ASEAN), World Health Assembly and Executive Board. Geneva. Fifty-Sixth Session (2003), Fifty-Seventh Session (2004), Fifty-Eighth Session (2005), Fifty-Ninth Session (2006), Sixtieth Session (2007), Sixty-First Session (2008), Sixty-Second Session (2009), Sixty-Third Session (2010). Files held with author.
World Health Organization (WHO). IHR Monitoring Framework. 2010–2016. www.who.int/gho/ihr/en/.
World Health Organization (WHO). *Weekly Epidemiological Record* (*WER*) Archives. 1996–2008. www.who.int/wer/archives/en/.
World Health Organization (WHO). *Weekly Epidemiological Record* (*WER*). 2009–2017. http://www.who.int/wer/en/.

Secondary Sources

Acharya, Amitav (2001). *Constructing a Security Community in Southeast Asia*. London: Routledge.
Acharya, Amitav (2004). "How Ideas Spread: Whose Norms Matter? Norm Localization and Institutional Change in Asian Regionalism." *International Organization* 58 (2): 239–275.

Acharya, Amitav (2006). "Securitization in Asia: Functional and Normative Implications." In Mely Cabellero-Anthony, Ralf Emmers, and Amitav Acharya (eds.), *Non-Traditional Security in Asia: Dilemmas in Securitization*, 247–250. Aldershot: Ashgate.

Acharya, Amitav (2007). "Human Security and Asian Regionalism: A Strategy of Localization." In Amitav Acharya and Evelyn Gosh (eds.), *Reassessing Security Cooperation in the Asia Pacific*, 237–252. Cambridge, MA: MIT Press.

Acharya, Amitav (2009). *Whose Ideas Matter? Agency and Power in Asian Regionalism*. Ithaca, NY: Cornell University Press.

African Health Stats (2016a). "Under-5 Mortality Rate." https://www.africanhealthstats.org/cms/.

African Health Stats (2016b). "Maternal Mortality Ratio." https://www.africanhealthstats.org/cms/.

Aldis, William (2008). "Health Security as a Public Health Concept: A Critical Analysis." *Health Policy and Planning* 23 (6): 369–375.

Alliance for Joint Evaluation Exercise (JEE) (2017). Alliance for JEE. https://www.jeealliance.org/.

Amaya, Ana B., Vincent Rollet, and Stephan Kingah (2015). "What's in a Word? The Framing of Health at the Regional Level: ASEAN, EU, SADC and UNASUR." *Global Social Policy* 15 (3): 229–260.

Anderson, Roy M., Christophe Fraser, Azra C. Ghani, Christl A. Donnelly, Steven Riley, Neil M. Ferguson, Gabriel M. Leung, Tai H. Lam, and Anthony J. Hedley (2003). "Epidemiology, Transmission Dynamics, and Control of SARS: The 2002–2003 Epidemic." In Angela R. McLean, Robert M. May, John Pattison, and Robin A. Weiss (eds.), *SARS: A Case Study in Emerging Infections*, 61–80. Oxford: Oxford University Press.

Arase, David (2010). "Non-Traditional Security in China-ASEAN Cooperation: The Institutionalization of Regional Security Cooperation and the Evolution of East Asian Regionalism." *Asian Survey* 50 (4): 808–833.

Association of Southeast Asian Nations (ASEAN) (2003a). "Joint Declaration Special ASEAN Leaders Meeting on Severe Acute Respiratory Syndrome (SARS), Bangkok, Thailand, 29 April." http://asean.org/joint-declaration-special-asean-leaders-meeting-on-severe-acute-respiratory-syndrome-sars-bangkok-thailand/.

Association of Southeast Asian Nations (ASEAN) (2003b). "Joint Statement of the Special ASEAN + 3 Health Ministers Meeting on Severe Acute Respiratory Syndrome (SARS), 'ASEAN Is a SARS Free Region,' Siem Reap, Cambodia, 10 June." http://asean.org/joint-statement-of-the-special-asean-3-health-ministers-meeting-on-severe-acute-respiratory-syndrome-sars-asean-is-a-sars-free-region-siem-reap-cambodia/.

Association of Southeast Asian Nations (ASEAN) (2006). "ASEAN Response to Combat Avian Influenza." ASEAN Secretariat. April. http://asean.org/?static_post=asean-response-to-combat-avian-influenza-by-asean-secretariat-3.

Association of Southeast Asian Nations (ASEAN) (2007). "2008 ASEAN Regional Strategy for the Progressive Control and Eradication of Highly Pathogenic Avian Influenza (2008–2010)." ASEAN Secretariat. http://asean.org/wp-content/uploads/images/ASEAN20Regional20Strategy20for20HPAI202008-2010.pdf.

Association of Southeast Asian Nations (ASEAN) (2008). The ASEAN Charter. Jakarta: ASEAN Secretariat. http://asean.org/wp-content/uploads/images/archive/publications/ASEAN-Charter.pdf.

Association of Southeast Asian Nations (ASEAN) (2009). *ASEAN Socio-cultural Community Blueprint*. Jakarta: ASEAN Secretariat.

Association of Southeast Asian Nations (ASEAN) (2011). "ASEAN Health Minister's Call for Action on the Control and Prevention of Dengue." Jakarta, 15 June. http://asean.org/jakarta-call-for-action-on-the-control-and-prevention-of-dengue-15-june-2011-jakarta-indonesia/.

Association of Southeast Asian Nations (ASEAN) (2012a). "ASEAN Health Profile: Regional Priorities and Programmes." Jakarta: ASEAN Secretariat.

Association of Southeast Asian Nations (ASEAN) (2012b). "ASEAN Medium Term Plan on Emerging Infectious Diseases (2012–2015) by ASEAN Expert Group on Communicable Diseases (AEGCD)." 11 July. On file with author.

Association of Southeast Asian Nations (ASEAN) (2014). "ASEAN Health Profile—Regional Priorities and Programmes for 2011–2015 (Updated Version)." September. On file with author.

Association of Southeast Asian Nations (ASEAN) (2016). *East Asia Summit Statement on Enhancing Regional Health Security relating to Infectious Diseases with Epidemic and Pandemic Potential.* 21 November. http://www.asean.org/storage/images/2015/November/10th-EAS -Outcome/EAS%20Statement%20on%20Enhancing%20Regional%20Health%20Security%20 -%20Final%2021%20November%202015.pdf.

ASEAN Health Ministers Meeting (AHMM) (2006). "Declaration of the 8th ASEAN Health Ministers Meeting: 'ASEAN Unity in Health Emergencies, 21 June, Yangon.'" http://www.asean .org/wp-content/uploads/images/2012/news/documents/Declaration%20of%20the%20 8th%20ASEAN%20Health%20Ministers%20Meeting.pdf.

ASEAN Health Ministers Meeting (AHMM) (2010). "Joint Statement of the 10th ASEAN Health Ministers Meeting, 22 July, Singapore." http://asean.org/?static_post=joint-statement-of-the -10th-asean-health-ministers.

ASEAN Plus Three (APT) (2007). *Protocol: Communication and Informational Sharing on Emerging Infectious Diseases in the ASEAN Plus Three Countries.* Jakarta: ASEAN Secretariat.

ASEAN Plus Three (APT) Health Ministers Meeting (2008). "Joint Statement of the Third ASEAN Plus Three Health Ministers Meeting, 10 October, Manila." http://asean.org/joint-statement -of-the-third-asean-plus-three-health-ministers-meeting-manila/.

ASEAN Plus Three (APT) Joint Statement (2004). "Joint Ministerial Statement on Avian Influenza, Bangkok, Thailand." http://www.asean.org/wp-content/uploads/2012/06/22206 .pdf.

ASEAN Secretariat (2012). "ASEAN Response to Combat Avian Influenza." In Heng-Lian Koh (ed.), *ASEAN Environmental Law, Policy and Governance: Selected Documents.* Singapore: World Scientific.

Australian Government (2017). *Evaluating a Decade of Australia's Efforts to Combat Pandemics and Emerging Infectious Diseases in Asia and the Pacific 2006–2015: Are Health Systems Stronger?* Office of Development Effectiveness, Department of Foreign Affairs and Trade. Canberra: Australian Government.

Ba, Alice D. (2009). *(Re)Negotiating East and Southeast Asia: Region, Regionalism, and ASEAN.* Stanford, CA: Stanford University Press.

Ba, Alice D. (2010). "Regional Security in East Asia: ASEAN's Value Added and Limitations." *Journal of Current Southeast Asian Affairs* 29 (3): 115–130.

Baker, Michael G. and David P. Fidler (2006). "Global Public Health Surveillance under New International Health Regulations." *Emerging Infectious Diseases* 12 (7): 1058–1065.

Bashford, Alison (2006). "'The Age of Universal Contagion': History, Disease and Globalization." In Alison Bashford (ed.), *Medicine at the Border: Disease, Globalization and Security, 1850 to the Present,* 1–17. Hampshire: Palgrave Macmillan.

Baum, Matthew A. and David A. Lake (2003). "The Political Economy of Growth: Democracy and Human Capital." *American Journal of Political Science* 47 (2): 333–347.

Bellamy Alex J. (2014). "The Other Asian Miracle? The Ending of Mass Atrocities in East Asia." *Global Change Peace and Security* 26 (1): 1–19.

Bennett, Carolyn (2009). "Lessons from SARS: Past Practice, Future Innovation." In Andrew F. Cooper and John J. Kirton (eds.), *Innovation in Global Health Governance,* 49–62. London: Routledge.

Besley, Timothy and Masayuki Kudamatsu (2006). "Health and Democracy." *American Economic Review* 96 (2): 313–318.

Borowy, Iris (2009). *Coming to Terms with World Health: The League of Nations Health Organisa-tion*. Frankfurt am Main: Peter Lang.

Boseley, Sarah (2015). "Ebola Is All but Over, but the Post-mortem Is Just Getting Started." *Guardian*, 30 September. https://www.theguardian.com/world/2015/sep/30/ebola-inquest-un-united-nations-world-health-organisation.

Briggs, Charles L., with Clara Mantini-Briggs (2003). *Stories in the Time of Cholera: Racial Profiling during a Medical Nightmare*. Berkeley: University of California Press.

Brown, Richard (2013). "Lessons from a Decade of Emerging Diseases: Towards Regional Public Health Security." *WHO South East Asia Journal of Public Health* 2 (2): 77–78.

Brown, Theodore M., Marcos Cueto, and Elizabeth Fee (2006). "The World Health Organization and the Transition From 'International' to 'Global' Public Health." *American Journal of Public Health* 96 (1): 62–72.

Brownstein, John S., Clark C. Freifeld, and Lawrence C. Madoff (2009). "Digital Disease Detection—Harnessing the Web for Public Health Surveillance." *New England Journal of Medicine* 360: 2153–2157.

Brownstein, John S., Clark C. Freifeld, Ben Y. Reis, and Kenneth D. Mandl (2008). "Surveillance sans Frontières: Internet-Based Emerging Infectious Disease Intelligence and the HealthMap Project." *Public Library of Science Medicine* 5 (7): e151.

Buzan, Barry, Ole Weaver, and Jaap de Wilde (1998). *Security: A New Framework for Analysis*. Boulder: Lynne Rienner.

Caballero-Anthony, Mely (2008). "Non-Traditional Security and Infectious Diseases in ASEAN: Going beyond the Rhetoric of Securitisation to Deeper Institutionalisation." *Pacific Review* 12 (4): 509–527.

Caballero-Anthony, Mely (2014). "Understanding ASEAN's Centrality: Bases and Prospects in an Evolving Regional Architecture." *Pacific Review* 27 (4): 563–584.

Caballero-Anthony, Mely, and Gianna Gayle Amul (2014). "Health and Human Security." In Simon Rushton and Jeremy Youde (eds.), *Routledge Handbook of Global Health Security*, 32–47. Abingdon: Routledge.

Caballero-Anthony, Mely, Alistair D. B. Cook, Gianna Gayle Herrera Amul, and Akanksha Sharma (2015). *Health Governance and Dengue in Southeast Asia*. NTS Report. Singapore: S. Rajaratnam School of International Studies.

Caballero-Anthony, Mely and Ralf Emmers (2006). "Understanding the Dynamics of Securitizing Non-Traditional Security." In Mely Cabellero-Anthony, Ralf Emmers, and Amitav Acharya (eds.), *Non-Traditional Security in Asia: Dilemmas in Securitization*. Aldershot: Ashgate.

Calain, Philippe (2007). "Exploring the International Arena of Global Public Health Surveillance." *Health Policy and Planning* 22 (1): 2–12.

Calain, Philippe and Caroline Abu Sa'Da (2015). "Coincident Polio and Ebola Crises Expose Similar Fault Lines in the Current Global Health Regime." *Conflict and Health* 9: 29–36.

Cash, Richard A. and Vasant Narasimhan (2000). "Impediments to Global Surveillance of Infectious Diseases: Consequences of Open Reporting in a Global Economy." *Bulletin of the World Health Organization* 78: 1358–1367.

Castillo-Salgado, Carlos (2010). "Trends and Directions of Global Public Health Surveillance." *Epidemiological Review* 32: 93–109.

Chalk, Peter (2006). "Disease and the Complex Processes of Securitization in the Asia Pacific." In Mely Cabellero-Anthony, Ralf Emmers, and Amitav Acharya (eds.), *Non-Traditional Security in Asia: Dilemmas in Securitization*, 112–135. Aldershot: Ashgate.

Chan, Emily H., Timothy F. Brewer, Lawrence C. Madoff, Marjorie P. Pollack, Amy L. Sonricker, Mikaela Keller, Clark C. Freifeld, Michael Blench, Abla Mawudeku, and John S. Brownstein (2010). "Global Capacity for Emerging Infectious Disease Detection." *Proceedings of the National Academy of Sciences* 107 (50): 21701–21706.

Chorev, Nitsan (2012). *The World Health Organization between North and South*. Ithaca, NY: Cornell University Press.

Coker, Richard J., Benjamin M. Hunter, James W. Rudge, Marco Liverani, and Piya Hanvoravongchai (2011). "Emerging Infectious Diseases in Southeast Asia: Regional Challenges to Control." *Lancet* 377 (9765): 599–609.

Collier, Nigel (2010). "What's Unusual in Online Disease Outbreak News?" *Journal of Biomedical Semantics* 1 (2): 1–18.

Collins, Alan (2013). "Norm Diffusion and ASEAN's Adoption and Adaption of Global HIV/AIDS Norms." *International Relations of the Asia-Pacific* 13 (3): 369–397.

Cortell, Andrew and Susan Peterson (2006). "Dutiful Agents, Rogue Agents, or Both? Staffing, Voting Rules, and Slack in the WHO and WTO." In Darren G. Hawkins, David A. Lake, Daniel L. Nielson, and Michael J. Tierney (eds.), *Delegation and Agency in International Organizations*, 225–280. Cambridge: Cambridge University Press.

Cotlear, Daniel, Somil Nagpal, Owen Smith, Ajay Tandon, and Rafael Cortez (2015). *Going Universal: How 24 Developing Countries Are Implementing Universal Health Coverage Reforms from the Bottom Up*. Washington, DC: World Bank.

Dafoe, Allan, John R. Oneal, and Bruce Russett (2013). "The Democratic Peace: Weighing the Evidence and Cautious Inference." *International Studies Quarterly* 57: 201–214.

Davies, Matthew (2013). "ASEAN and Human Rights Norms: Constructivism, Rational Choice, and the Action-Identity Gap." *International Relations of the Asia-Pacific* 13 (2): 207–231.

Davies, Sara (2007). *Legitimising Rejection: International Refugee Law in Southeast Asia*. Refugees and Human Rights Series 13. Leiden: Martinus Nijhoff.

Davies, Sara E. (2012). "The International Politics of Disease Reporting: Towards Post-Westphalianism?" *International Politics* 49 (5): 591–613.

Davies, Sara E. (2017). "Mind the Human Rights Gap in Outbreak Response." *Medical Law Review* 25 (2): 270–292.

Davies, Sara E., Adam Kamradt-Scott, and Simon Rushton (2015). *Disease Diplomacy*. Baltimore: Johns Hopkins University Press.

Davies, Sara E., Kimberly Nackers, and Sarah Teitt (2014). "Women, Peace and Security as an ASEAN Priority." *Australian Journal of International Affairs* 68 (3): 333–355.

Davies, Sara E. and Jeremy Youde (2012). "The IHR (2005), Disease Surveillance, and the Individual in Global Health Politics." *International Journal of Human Rights* 17 (1): 133–151.

Desclaux Alice, Moustapha Diop, and Stephane Doyon (2017). "Fear and Containment: Contact Follow-Up Perceptions and Social Effetcs in Senegal and Guinea." In Michiel Hofman and Sokhieng Au (eds.), *The Politics of Fear: Médecins sans Frontières and the West African Ebola Epidemic*. Oxford: Oxford University Press.

Doner, Richard F., Bryan K. Ritchie, and Dan Slater (2005). "Systemic Vulnerability and the Origins of Developmental States: Northeast and Southeast Asia in Comparative Perspective." *International Organization* 59: 327–361.

Dosch, Jörn (2008). "ASEAN's Reluctant Liberal Turn and the Thorny Road to Democracy Promotion." *Pacific Review* 21 (4): 527–545.

Ear, Sophal (2010). "Cambodia's Patient Zero: Global and National Responses to Highly Pathogenic Avian Influenza." In Ian Scoones (ed.), *Avian Influenza: Science, Policy and Politics*, 65–92. London: Earthscan.

Ear, Sophal (2012). *Aid Dependence in Cambodia: How Foreign Assistance Undermines Democracy*. New York: Columbia University Press.

Elbe, Stefan (2010). "Haggling over Viruses: The Downside Risks of Securitizing Infectious Disease." *Health Policy and Planning* 25 (6): 476–485.

Elbe, Stefan (2011). "Should Health Professionals Play the Global Health Security Card?" *Lancet* 378 (9787): 220–221.

Enemark, Christian (2007). *Disease and Security: Natural Plagues and Biological Weapons in East Asia*. Abingdon: Routledge.

Enemark, Christian (2017). *Biosecurity Dilemmas: Dreaded Diseases, Ethical Responses, and the Health of Nations*. Washington, DC: Georgetown University Press.

Fidler, David P. (1999). *International Law and Infectious Diseases*. Oxford: Oxford University Press.

Fidler, David P. (2004a). *SARS, Governance and the Globalization of Disease*. Hampshire: Palgrave Macmillan.

Fidler, David P. (2004b). "Germs, Governance, and Global Public Health in the Wake of SARS." *Journal of Clinical Investigation* 113 (6): 799–804.

Fidler, David P. (2005). "From International Sanitary Conventions to Global Health Security: The New International Health Regulations." *Chinese Journal of International Law* 4 (2): 325–392.

Fidler, David P. (2013). "Asia and Global Health Governance: Power, Principles, and Practice." In Kelley Lee, Tikki Pang, and Yeling Tan (eds.), *Asia's Role in Governing Global Health*, 98–214. Abingdon, UK: Routledge.

Fidler, David P. (2015). "Ebola Report Misses Mark on International Health Regulations." 17 July. https://www.chathamhouse.org/expert/comment/ebola-report-misses-mark-international-health-regulations.

Fidler, David P. and Lawrence O. Gostin (2008). *Biosecurity in the Global Age: Biological Weapons, Public Health, and the Rule of Law*. Stanford, CA: Stanford University Press.

Field, Emma and Takeshi Kasai (2010). "Western Pacific Surveillance and Response: A Journal to Reflect the Needs of Our Region." *Western Pacific Surveillance and Response Journal* 1 (1): 1–2.

Finnemore, Martha and Kathryn Sikkink (1998). "International Norm Dynamics and Political Change." *International Organization* 52 (4): 887–917.

Fischer, Julie and Rebecca Katz (2013). "Moving Forward to 2014: Global IHR (2005) Implementation." *Biosecurity and Bioterrorism: Biodefense Strategy Practice and Science* 11 (2): 153–156.

Fluss, S. S. and Frank Gutteridge (1990). "Some Contributions of the World Health Organization to Legislation." In Thomas A. Lambo and Stacey B. Day (eds.), *Issues in Contemporary International Health*. Boston: Springer.

Food and Agriculture Organization and World Health Organization (FAO/WHO) (2004). "Unprecedented Spread of Avian Influenza Requires Broad Collaboration, FAO/OIE/WHO Call for International Assistance." 27 January. http://www.who.int/mediacentre/news/releases/2004/pr7/en/.

Foot, Rosemary (2014). "Social Boundaries in Flux: Secondary Regional Organizations as a Reflection of Regional International Society." In Barry Buzan and Yongjin Zhang (eds.), *Contesting International Society in Asia*, 247–250. Cambridge: Cambridge University Press.

Forster, Paul (2010). "On a Wing and a Prayer: Avian Influenza in Indonesia." In Ian Scoones (ed.), *Avian Influenza: Science, Policy and Politics*, 131–168. London: Earthscan.

Freifeld, Clark C., K. D. Mandl, B. Y. Reis, and J. S. Brownstein (2008). "HealthMap: Global Infectious Disease Monitoring through Automated Classification and Visualization of Internet Media Reports." *Journal of American Medical Information Association* 15 (2): 150–157.

Gerard, Kelly (2013). "From the ASEAN People's Assembly to the ASEAN Civil Society Conference: The Boundaries of Civil Society Advocacy." *Contemporary Politics* 19 (4): 411–426.

Gevrek, Deniz and Karen Middleton (2016). "Globalization and Women's and Girls' Health in 192 UN-Member Countries: Convention on the Elimination of All Forms of Discrimination against Women." *International Journal of Social Economics* 43 (7): 692–721.

Ghobarah, Hazem Adam, Paul Huth, and Bruce Russett (2004). "The Post-war Public Health Effects of Civil Conflict." *Social Science & Medicine* 59 (4): 869–884.

Giorgetti, Chiara (2010). *A Principled Approach to State Failure: International Community Actions in Emergency Situations.* Boston: Brill.

Giorgetti, Chiara (2012). "International Health Emergencies in Failed and Failing States." *Georgetown Journal of International Law* 44: 1347–1386.

Global Health Security Agenda (GHSA) (2016). *Advancing the Global Health Security Agenda: Progress and Early Impact from US Investment.* Washington, DC: Office of the President of the United States of America, Department of Health and Human Services, Centers for Disease Control and Prevention, USAID, Department of Defense, USDA, Department of Justice, Department of Homeland Security.

Goh, Evelyn (2013). *The Struggle for Order: Hegemony, Hierarchy, and Transition in Post–Cold War East Asia.* Oxford: Oxford University Press.

Goh, Evelyn (2014). "Southeast Asia's Evolving Security Relations and Strategies." In Sadia M. Pekkanen, John Ravenhill, and Rosemary Foot (eds.), *The Oxford Handbook of the International Relations of Asia,* 462–480. New York: Oxford University Press.

Goldsmith, Benjamin E. (2013). "Different in Asia? Developmental States, Trade, and International Conflict Onset and Escalation." *International Relations of the Asia-Pacific* 13 (2): 175–205.

Goldsmith, Benjamin E. (2014). "The East Asian Peace as a Second-Order Diffusion Effect." *International Studies Review* 16 (2): 275–289.

Gostin, Lawrence O. (2012). "A Framework Convention on Global Health: Health for All, Justice for All." *Journal of the American Medical Association* 307: 2087–2092.

Gostin, Lawrence O. and Eric A. Friedman (2015). "A Retrospective and Prospective Analysis of the West African Ebola Virus Disease Epidemic: Robust National Health Systems at the Foundation and an Empowered WHO at the Apex." *Lancet* 385 (9980): 1902–1909.

Gostin, Lawrence O. and Rebecca Katz (2016). "The International Health Regulations: The Governing Framework for Global Health Security." *Milbank Quarterly* 94: 264–313.

Gostin, Lawrence O., Oyewale Tomori, Suwit Wibulpolprasert, Ashish K. Jha, Julio Frenk, Sueri Moon, Joy Phumaphi, Peter Piot, Barbara Stocking, Victor J. Dzau, and Gabriel M. Leung (2016). "Toward a Common Secure Future: Four Global Commissions in the Wake of Ebola." *Public Library of Science Medicine* 13 (5): 1–15.

Grein, Thomas W., Kamara O. Kande-Bure, Guénaël Rodier, Aileen J. Plant, Patrick Bovier, Michael J. Ryan, Takaaki Ohyama, and David L. Heymann (2000). "Rumors of Disease in the Global Village: Outbreak Verification." *Emerging Infectious Diseases* 6 (2): 97–102.

Grépin, Karen A. and Kim Y. Dionne (2013). "Democratization and Universal Health Coverage: A Comparison of the Experiences of Ghana, Kenya, and Senegal." *Global Health Governance* 6 (2): 1–27.

Gresham, Louise S., Mark S. Smolinski, Rapeepong Suphanchaimat, Ann Marie Kimball, and Suwit Wibulpolprasert (2013). "Creating a Global Dialogue on Infectious Disease Surveillance: Connecting Organizations for Regional Disease Surveillance (CORDS)." *Emerging Health Threats Journal* 6: 1–7.

Gronke, Paul (2015). "The Politics and Policy of Ebola." *PS: Political Science & Politics,* 48 (1): 3–18.

Haacke, Jürgen (2009). "Myanmar, the Responsibility to Protect, and the Need for Practical Assistance." *Global Responsibility to Protect* 1 (2): 156–184.

Haacke, Jürgen and Noel M. Morada (2010). "The ASEAN Regional Forum and Cooperative Security: Introduction." In Jürgen Haacke and Noel M. Morada (eds.), *Cooperative Security in the Asia-Pacific: The ASEAN Regional Forum,* 1–12. Asian Security Studies. Oxford: Routledge, Oxford.

Haacke, Jürgen and Paul D. Williams (2008). "Regional Arrangements, Securitization, and Transnational Security Challenges: The African Union and the Association of Southeast Asian Nations Compared." *Security Studies* 17 (4): 775–809.

Haas, Peter M. (1992). "Introduction: Epistemic Communities and International Policy Coordination." *International Organization* 46 (1): 1–35.

Hameiri, Shahar (2014). "Avian Influenza, 'Viral Sovereignty,' and the Politics of Health Security in Indonesia." *Pacific Review* 27 (3): 333–356.

Hardiman, Maxwell Charles (2012). "World Health Organization Perspective on Implementation of International Health Regulations." *Emerging Infectious Diseases* 18 (7): 1041–1046.

Hartley, David, Noele Nelson, Ronald Walters, Ray Arthur, Roman Yangarber, Larry Madoff, Jens Linge, Abla Mawudeku, Nigel Collier, John Brownstein, Germain Thinus, and Nigel Lightfoot (2010). "The Landscape of International Event-Based Biosurveillance." *Emerging Health Threats Journal* 3: e3.

Heffelfinger, James D., Xi Li, Nyambat Batmunkh, Varja Grabovac, Sergey Diorditsa, Jayantha B. Liyanage, Sirima Pattamadilok, Sunil Bahl, Kirsten S. Vannice, Terri B. Hyde, Susan Y. Chu, Kimberley K. Fox, Susan L. Hills, and Anthony A. Marfin (2017). "Japanese Encephalitis: Surveillance and Immunization in Asia and the Western Pacific, 2016." *WHO Weekly Epidemiological Record* 92 (23): 323–331.

Hegre, Håvard (2014). "Democracy and Armed Conflict." *Journal of Peace Research* 51 (2): 159–172.

Herrington, Jonathan (2010). "Securitization of Infectious Diseases in Vietnam: The Cases of HIV and Avian Influenza." *Health Policy and Planning* 25 (6): 467–475.

Heymann, David L. (2006). "SARS and Emerging Infectious Diseases: A Challenge to Place Global Solidarity above National Sovereignty." *Annals, Academy of Medicine, Singapore* 35: 350–353.

Heymann, David L. and Guénaël R. Rodier (2004). "Global Surveillance, National Surveillance, and SARS." *Emerging Infectious Diseases* 10 (2): 173–175.

Heymann, David L. and Alison West (2014). "Emerging Infections: Threats to Health and Economic Security." In Simon Rushton and Jeremy Youde (eds.), *Routledge Handbook of Global Health Security*, 92–104. Abingdon: Routledge.

Heywood, Alison and Moussavi, Saba (2010). *Independent Evaluation of the Asia Pacific Strategy for Emerging Diseases (APSED)*. Final report. 17 June. On file with author.

High Level Panel on the Global Response to Health Crises (2016). *Protecting Humanity from Future Health Crises*, 25 January. www.un.org/News/dh/infocus/HLP/2016-02-05_Final_Report _Global_Response_to_Health_Crises.pdf.

Hofman, Michiel and Sokhieng Au (2017). *The Politics of Fear: Médecins sans Frontières and the West African Ebola Epidemic*. Oxford: Oxford University Press.

Horby, Peter W., Dirk Pfeiffer, and Hitoshi Oshitani (2013). "Prospects for Emerging Infections in East and Southeast Asia 10 Years after Severe Acute Respiratory Syndrome." *Emerging Infectious Diseases* 19 (6): 853–860.

House of Lords (2008). *Diseases Know No Frontiers: How Effective Are Intergovernmental Organisations in Controlling Their Spread?* Select Committee on Intergovernmental Organizations, 1st Report Session of 2007–2008, HL Paper 143–II, 21 July. Westminster: UK Government.

Ijaz, Kashef, Eric Kasowski, Ray R. Arthur, Frederick J. Angulo, and Scott F. Dowell (2012). "International Health Regulations—What Gets Measured Gets Done." *Emerging Infectious Diseases* 18 (7): 1054–1057.

Institute for Health Metrics and Evaluation (IHME) (2010). *Financing Global Health 2010: Development Assistance and Country Spending in Economic Uncertainty*. Seattle, WA: IHME.

Institute for Health Metrics and Evaluation (IHME) (2013). *GBD 2010 Life Expectancy 1990–2010*. Seattle, WA: IHME. http://ghdx.healthdata.org/record/global-burden-disease-study-2010-gbd -2010-life-expectancy-and-healthy-life-expectancy-1970.

International Crisis Group (ICG) (2012). *Myanmar: Storm Clouds on the Horizon*. Asia Report 238. 12 Nov. https://www.crisisgroup.org/asia/south-east-asia/myanmar/myanmar-storm -clouds-horizon.

International Crisis Group (ICG) (2015). *The Politics behind the Ebola Crisis.* 28 October. https://www.crisisgroup.org/africa/west-africa/politics-behind-ebola-crisis.

International Working Group on Financial Preparedness (2017). *From Panic and Neglect to Investing in Health Security: Financing Pandemic Preparedness at a National Level.* Washington, DC: World Bank.

Iqbal, Zaryab (2010). *War and the Health of Nations.* Stanford, CA: Stanford University Press.

Johnston, Alastair Iain (2012). "What (If Anything) Does East Asia Tell Us about International Relations Theory?" *Annual Review of Political Science* 15: 53–78.

Jones, Kate E., Nikkita G. Patel, Marc A. Levy, Adam Storeygard, Deborah Balk, John L. Gittleman, and Peter Daszak (2008). "Global Trends in Emerging Infectious Diseases." *Nature* 451: 990–993.

Jones, Lee (2012). *ASEAN, Sovereignty and Intervention in Southeast Asia.* Basingstoke: Palgrave Macmillan.

Justesen, Mogens K. (2012). "Democracy, Dictatorship, and Disease: Political Regimes and HIV/AIDS." *European Journal of Political Economy* 28 (3): 373–389.

Kalin, Walter (2015). "Ritual and Ritualism at the Universal Periodic Review: A Preliminary Appraisal." In Hilary Charlesworth and Emma Larking (eds.), *Human Rights and the Universal Periodic Review*, 25–41. Cambridge: Cambridge University Press.

Kamradt-Scott, Adam (2010). "The WHO Secretariat, Norm Entrepreneurship, and Global Disease Outbreak Control." *Journal of International Organizations Studies* 1 (1): 72–89.

Kamradt-Scott, Adam (2014). "Health, Security and Diplomacy in Historical Perspective." In Simon Rushton and Jeremy Youde (eds.), *Routledge Handbook of Global Health Security*, 189–200. Abingdon: Routledge.

Kamradt-Scott, Adam (2015). *Managing Global Health Security: The World Health Organization and Disease Outbreak Control.* Hampshire: Palgrave Macmillan.

Kamradt-Scott, Adam (2016). "WHO's to Blame? The World Health Organization and the 2014 Ebola Outbreak in West Africa." *Third World Quarterly* 37 (3): 401–418.

Kamradt-Scott, Adam, Kelley Lee, and Jingying Xu (2013). "The International Health Regulations (2005): Asia's Contribution to a Global Health Governance Framework." In Kelley Lee, Tikki Pang, and Yeling Tan (eds.), *Asia's Role in Governing Global Health*, 83–98. Abingdon, UK: Routledge.

Kasolo, Francis, Zabulon Yoti, Nathan Bakyaita, Peter Gaturuku, Rebecca Katz, Julie E. Fischer, and Helen N. Perry (2013). "IDSR as a Platform for Implementing IHR in African Countries." *Biosecurity and Bioterrorism* 11 (3): 163–169.

Katz, Rebecca (2009). "Use of the Revised International Health Regulations during Influenza A (H1N1) Epidemic, 2009." *Emerging Infectious Diseases* 15 (8): 1166.

Katz, Rebecca and Julie Fischer (2010). "The Revised International Health Regulations: A Framework for Global Pandemic Response." *Global Health Governance* 3 (2): 1–18.

Katz, Rebecca, Vibhuti Haté, Sarah Kornblet, and Julie E. Fischer (2012). "Costing Framework for International Health Regulations (2005)." *Emerging Infectious Disease* 18 (7): 1121–1127.

Kimball, Ann Marie, Melinda Moore, Howard Matthew French, Yuzo Arima, Kumnuan Ungchusak, Suwit Wibulpolprasert, Terence Taylor, Sok Touch, and Alex Leventhal (2008). "Regional Infectious Disease Surveillance Networks and Their Potential to Facilitate the Implementation of the International Health Regulations." *Medical Clinics* 92 (6): 1459–1471.

Kivimäki, Timo (2011). "East Asian Relative Peace and the ASEAN Way." *International Relations of the Asia-Pacific* 11 (1): 57–85.

Kivimäki, Timo (2012). "Sovereignty, Hegemony, and Peace in Western Europe and in East Asia." *International Relations of the Asia-Pacific* 12 (3): 419–447.

Klobentz, Gregory D. (2010). "Biosecurity Reconsidered: Calibrating Biological Threats and Responses." *International Security* 34 (4): 96–132.

Klomp, Jeroen and Jakob de Haan (2009). "Is the Political System Really Related to Health?" *Social Science & Medicine* 69 (1): 36–46.

Kluberg, Sheryl A., Sumiko R. Mekaru, David J. McIver, Lawrence C. Madoff, Adam W. Crawley, Mark S. Smolinski, and John S. Brownstein (2016). "Global Capacity for Emerging Infectious Disease Detection, 1996–2014." *Emerging Infectious Diseases* 22 (10).

Koblentz, Gregory D. (2012). "From Biodefense to Biosecurity." *International Affairs* 88 (1): 131–148.

Kohl, Katrin S., Cody Thornton, Jose Fernandez, Nicki Pesik, Francisco Alvarado-Ramy, Martin Cetron, and Ray Arthur (2014). "Notifications of Public Health Events under the International Health Regulations—5 Year U.S. Experience." *Online Journal of Public Health Informatics* 6 (1): e104.

Kool Jakob L., Beverley Paterson, Boris I. Pavlin, David Durrheim, Jennie Musto, and Anthony Kolbe (2012). "Pacific-Wide Simplified Syndromic Surveillance for Early Warning of Outbreaks." *Global Public Health* 7 (7): 670–681.

Kruk, Margaret E., Michael Myers, S. Tornorlah Varpilah, and Bernice T. Dahn (2015). "What Is a Resilient Health System? Lessons from Ebola." *Lancet* 385 (9980): 1910–1912.

Kumaresan, Jacob and Suvi Huikuri (2015). "Strengthening Regional Cooperation, Coordination, and Response to Health Concerns in the ASEAN Region: Status, Challenges, and Ways Forward." ERIA Discussion Paper Series, September.

Lake, David A. and Matthew A. Baum (2001). "The Invisible Hand of Democracy." *Comparative Political Studies* 34 (6): 587–621.

Lamy, Marie and Kai Hong Phua (2012). "Southeast Asian Cooperation in Health: A Comparative Perspective on Regional Health Governance in ASEAN and the EU." *Asia Europe Journal* 10 (4): 233–250.

Lancet (2007). "International Health Regulations—the Challenges Ahead." *Lancet* 369 (9575): 1763.

Lee, Kelley (2008). *The World Health Organization*. Global Institutions Series. Abingdon: Routledge.

Lee, Kelley and David P. Fidler (2007). "Avian and Pandemic Influenza: Progress and Problems with Global Health Governance." *Global Public Health* 2 (3): 215–234.

Leifer, Michael (1989). "The Role and Paradox of ASEAN." In Michael Leifer (ed.), *The Balance of Power in East Asia*, 119–131. Basingstoke: Palgrave Macmillan.

Li, Ailan (2013). "Implementing the International Health Regulations (2005) in the World Health Organization Western Pacific Region." *Western Pacific Surveillance and Response Journal* 4 (3): 1–3.

Li, Ailan and Takeshi Kasai (2011). "The Asia Pacific Strategy for Emerging Diseases: A Strategy for Regional Health Security." *Western Pacific Surveillance and Response Journal* 2 (1): 6–9.

Linge, Jens P., R. Steinberger, T. P. Weber, R. Yangarber, E. van der Goot, D. H. al Khudhairy, and N. I. Stilianakis (2009). "Internet Surveillance Systems for Early Alerting of Health Threats." *European Surveillance* 14 (13): 19162.

Liverani, Marco and Richard Coker (2012). "Protecting Europe from Diseases: From the International Sanitary Conferences to the ECDC." *Journal of Health Politics, Policy and Law* 37 (6): 913–932.

Mack, Eric (2006). "The World Health Organization's New International Health Regulations: Incursion on State Sovereignty and Ill-Fated Response to Global Health Issues." *Chicago Journal of International Law* 7 (1): 365–377.

Mackenbach, Johan P., Yannan Hu, and Caspar W. N. Looman (2013). "Democratization and Life Expectancy in Europe, 1960–2008." *Social Science & Medicine* 93: 166–175.

Mackenbach, Johan P. and Martin McKee (2015). "Government, Politics and Health Policy: A Quantitative Analysis of 30 European Countries." *Health Policy* 119 (10): 1298–1308.

Mackenzie, John S. and Angela Merianos (2013). "The Legacies of SARS—International Preparedness and Readiness to Respond to Future Threats in the Western Pacific Region." *Western Pacific Surveillance and Response Journal* 4 (3): 4–8.

Madoff, Lawrence C. and John P. Woodall (2005). "The Internet and the Global Monitoring of Emerging Diseases: Lessons from the First 10 Years of ProMED-mail." *Archives of Medical Research* 36: 724–730.

Mahapatra, Tanmay, Sanchita Mahapatra, Giridhara R. Babu, Weiming Tang, Barnali Banerjee, Umakanta Mahapatra, and Aritra Das (2014). "Cholera Outbreaks in South and Southeast Asia: Descriptive Analysis, 2003–2012." *Japanese Journal of Infectious Diseases* 67 (3): 145–156.

Mahbubani, Kishore (2008). *The New Asian Hemisphere: The Irresistible Shift of Global Power to the East*. New York: Public Affairs.

Maier-Knapp, Naila (2011). "Regional and Interregional Integrative Dynamics of ASEAN and EU in Response to the Avian Influenza." *Asia Europe Journal* 8 (4): 541–554.

Marshall, Monty and Ted Gurr (2014). "Polity IV Project: Political Regime Characteristics and Transitions, 1800–2013." June. http://www.systemicpeace.org/polity/polity4.htm.

McInnes, Colin (2015). "WHO's Next? Changing Authority in Global Health Governance after Ebola." *International Affairs* 91 (6): 1299–1316.

McInnes, Colin J. and Kelley Lee (2006). "Health, Security and Foreign Policy." *Review of International Studies* 32 (1): 5–23.

McInnes, Colin and Anne Roemer-Mahler (2017). "From Security to Risk: Reframing Global Health Threats." *International Affairs* 93 (6), 1313–1338.

McKenna, Maryn (2010). "Southeast Asia Aims to Eradicate H5N1 by 2020." CIDRAP. 28 April. http://www.cidrap.umn.edu/news-perspective/2010/04/southeast-asia-aims-eradicate-h5n1-2020.

Moon, Suerie, Devi Sridhar, Muhammed A. Pate, et al. (2015). "Will Ebola Change the Game? Ten Essential Reforms before the Next Pandemic: The Report of the Harvard LSHTM Independent Panel on the Global Response to Ebola." *Lancet* 386 (10009): 2204–2221.

Moore, Melinda, Bill Gelfield, Adeyemi Okunogbe, and Christopher Paul (2016). *Identifying Future Hot Spots: Infectious Disease Vulnerability Index*. Washington, DC: RAND.

Morada, Noel M. (2009). "The ASEAN Charter and the Promotion of R2P in Southeast Asia: Challenges and Constraints." *Global Responsibility to Protect* 1 (2): 185–207.

Morris, R. S. and R. Jackson (2005). "Epidemiology of H5N1 Avian Influenza in Asia and Implications for Regional Control." Commissioned Report for Food and Agriculture Organization of the United Nations. April. Rome: Food and Agriculture Organization of the United Nations. http://www.fao.org/docs/eims/upload/246974/aj122e00.pdf.

Mousseau, Michael, Håvard Hegre, and John R. Oneal (2003). "How the Wealth of Nations Conditions the Liberal Peace." *European Journal of International Relations* 9 (2): 277–314.

Mulbah, Edward, Nontobeko Zondi, and Lesley Connolly (2015). "Picking Up the Pieces: Liberia's Peacebuilding Efforts Post-Ebola." ACCORD Policy Practice Brief 35, 24 August. http://www.accord.org.za/publication/picking-up-the-pieces/.

Muntaner, Carles (2013). "Democracy, Authoritarianism, Political Conflict, and Population Health: A Global, Comparative, and Historical Approach." *Social Science and Medicine* 86: 107–112.

Murray, Philomena (2014). "Europe and the World: The Problem of the Fourth Wall in EU-ASEAN Norms Promotion." *Journal of Contemporary European Studies* 23 (2): 238–252.

Narine, Shaun (2002). *Explaining ASEAN: Regionalism in Southeast Asia*. Boulder: Lynne Rienner.

O'Malley, Peter, John Rainford, and Alison Thompson (2009). "Transparency during Public Health Emergencies: From Rhetoric to Reality." *Bulletin of the World Health Organization* 87: 614–618.

Oneal, John R. and Bruce M. Russett (1997). "The Classical Liberals Were Right: Democracy, Interdependence, and Conflict, 1950–1985." *International Studies Quarterly* 41: 267–293.

Ottersen, Ole P., J. Dasgupta, C. Blouin, et al. (2014). "The Political Origins of Health Inequity: Prospects for Change." *Lancet* 383 (2014): 630–667.

Oxfam International (2015). "Improving International Governance for Global Health Emergencies: Lessons from the Ebola Crisis." Oxfam Discussion Paper, January. https://www.oxfam .org/sites/www.oxfam.org/files/file_attachments/dp-governance-global-health-emergencies -ebola-280115-en.pdf.

Paterson, Beverley J., Jacob L. Kool, David N. Durrheim, and Boris Pavlin (2012). "Sustaining Surveillance: Evaluating Syndromic Surveillance in the Pacific." *Global Public Health* 7 (7): 682–694.

Patterson, Andrew C. (2017). "Not All Built the Same? A Comparative Study of Electoral Systems and Population Health." *Health & Place* 47: 90–99.

Paxton, Nathan (2015). "Doctors Blame the WHO and the U.N. for Failing to Fight Ebola: Here's Why They're Wrong." Monkey Cage. *Washington Post*, 20 January. https://www.washingtonpost .com/news/monkey-cage/wp/2015/01/20/doctors-blame-the-who-and-the-u-n-for-failing -to-fight-ebola-heres-why-theyre-wrong/?utm_term=.79635cf5babd.

Pega, Frank, Ichiro Kawachi, Kumanan Rasanathan, and Olle Lundberg (2015). "Politics, Policies and Population Health: A Commentary on Mackenbach, Hu and Looman (2013)." *Social Science & Medicine* 93: 176–179.

Perlo-Freeman, Sam (2012). "Budgetary Priorities in Latin America: Military, Health and Education Spending." *SIPRI Insights on Peace and Security* (2011/12). http://books.sipri.org/product _info?c_product_id=436.

Phommasack, Bounlay, Chuleeporn Jiraphongsa, Moe Ko Oo, Katherine C. Bond, Natalie Phaholyothin, Rapeepong Suphanchaimat, Kumnuan Ungchusak, and Sarah B. Macfarlane (2013). "Mekong Basin Disease Surveillance (MBDS): A Trust-Based Network." *Emerging Health Threats Journal* 6: 19944.

Pitsuwan, Surin (2011). "Challenges in Infection in ASEAN." *Lancet* 377 (9766): 619–621.

Plotkin, Bruce J. (2007). "Human Rights and Other Provisions in the Revised International Health Regulations (2005)." *Public Health* 121: 840–845.

Plotkin, Bruce J. and Max. C. Hardiman (2013). "Infectious Disease Surveillance and the International Health Regulations." In N. M. M'ikanatha, R. Lynfield, C. A. Van Beneden, and H. de Valk (eds.), *Infectious Disease Surveillance.* 2nd ed. Oxford: John Wiley & Sons.

Plümper, Thomas and Eric Neumayer (2006). "The Unequal Burden of War: The Effect of Armed Conflict on the Gender Gap in Life Expectancy." *International Organization* 60: 723–754.

Price-Smith, Andrew T. (2002). *The Health of Nations.* Cambridge, MA: MIT Press.

Price-Smith, Andrew T. (2009). *Contagion and Chaos.* Cambridge, MA: MIT Press.

Ramiah, Ilavenil (2006). "Securitizing the AIDS Issue in Asia." In Mely Cabellero-Anthony, Ralf Emmers, and Amitav Acharya (eds.), *Non-Traditional Security in Asia: Dilemmas in Securitization*, 136–167. Aldershot: Ashgate.

Rockers, Peter C., Margaret E. Kruk, and Megan J. Laugesen (2012). "Perceptions of the Health System and Public Trust in Government in Low- and Middle-Income Countries: Evidence from the World Health Surveys." *Journal of Health Politics, Policy and Law* 37 (3): 405–437.

Rod, E. G. and N. B. Weildman (2015). "Empowering Activists or Autocrats? The Internet in Authoritarian Regimes." *Journal of Peace Research* 52 (3): 338–351.

Rodier, Guénaël R. (2007). "New Rules on International Public Health Security." *Bulletin of the World Health Organization* 85 (6): 428–431.

Ross, Michael (2006). "Is Democracy Good for the Poor?" *American Journal of Political Science* 50 (4): 860–874.

Ruger, Jennifer Prah (2005). "Democracy and Health." *QJM: Monthly Journal of the Association of Physicians* 98 (4): 299–304.

Safman, Rachel A. (2010). "Avian Influenza Control in Thailand: Balancing the Interests of Different Poultry Producers." In Ian Scoones (ed.), *Avian Influenza: Science, Policy and Politics*, 169–206. London: Earthscan.

Salomon, Joshua A., H. Wang, M. K. Freeman, T. Vos, A. D. Flaxman, A. D. Lopez, and C. J. L. Murray (2012). "Healthy Life Expectancy for 187 Countries, 1990–2010: A Systematic Analysis for the Global Burden Disease Study 2010." *Lancet* 380: 2144–2162.

Sandholtz, Wayne (2008). "Dynamics of International Norm Change." *European Journal of International Relations* 14 (1): 101–131.

Schneider, Gerald (2013). "Peace through Globalization and Capitalism? Prospects of Two Liberal Propositions." *Journal of Peace Research* 51 (2): 173–183.

Sengupta, Somini (2015). "Effort on Ebola Hurt WHO Chief." *New York Times*, 6 January. https://www.nytimes.com/2015/01/07/world/leader-of-world-health-organization-defends-ebola-response.html?_r=0.

Shiffman, Jeremy (2006). "Donor Funding Priorities for Communicable Disease Control in the Developing World." *Health Policy and Planning* 21 (6): 411–420.

Smith, Frank (2012). "Insights into Surveillance from the Influenza Virus and Benefit Sharing Controversy." *Global Change, Peace and Security* 24 (1): 71–81.

Spiegel, Paul B., Anne Rygaard Bennedsen, Johanna Claass, Laurie Bruns, Njogu Patterson, Dieudonne Yiweza, and Marian Schilperoord (2007). "Prevalence of HIV Infection in Conflict-Affected and Displaced People in Seven Sub-Saharan African Countries: A Systematic Review." *Lancet* 369 (9580): 2187–2195.

Sridhar, Devi and Lawrence O. Gostin (2011). "Reforming the World Health Organization." Georgetown Law Faculty Publications and Other Works. 623. https://scholarship.law.georgetown.edu/facpub/623.

Sridhar, Devi, Janelle Winters, and Eleanor Strong (2017). "World Bank's Financing, Priorities, and Lending Structures for Global Health." *British Medical Journal* 358 (3339): 1–4.

Stevenson, Michael A. and Andrew F. Cooper (2009). "Overcoming Constraints of State Sovereignty: Global Health Governance in Asia." *Third World Quarterly* 30 (7): 1379–1394.

Stubbs, Richard (2014). "ASEAN's Leadership in East Asian Region-Building: Strength in Weakness." *Pacific Review* 27 (4): 523–541.

Supari, Siti Fadilah (2008). *It's Time for the World to Change in the Spirit of Dignity, Equity, and Transparency*. Jakarta: PT Sulaksana Warinsa Indonesia.

Tan, Hsien-Li (2011). *The ASEAN Intergovernmental Commission on Human Rights: Institutionalising Human Rights in Southeast Asia*. Cambridge: Cambridge University Press.

Tang, Chih-Mao (2012). "Southeast Asian Peace Revisited: A Capitalist Trajectory." *International Relations of the Asia-Pacific* 12 (3): 389–417.

Tarling, Nicholas (2006). "Regionalism in Southeast Asia: To Foster the Political Will." Abingdon: Routledge.

Taydas, Zeynep and Dursun Peksen (2012). "Can States Buy Peace? Social Welfare Spending and Civil Conflicts." *Journal of Peace Research* 49 (2): 273–287.

Taylor, Allyn L. (2002). "Global Governance, International Health Law and WHO: Looking Towards the Future." *Bulletin of the World Health Organization* 80 (12): 975–980.

Thakur, Ramesh and Thomas G. Weiss (2009). "United Nations 'Policy': An Argument with Three Illustrations." *International Studies Perspectives* 10 (1): 18–35.

Thomas, Nicholas (2006). "The Regionalization of Avian Influenza in East Asia: Responding to the Next Pandemic(?)." *Asian Survey* 46 (6): 917–936.

United Nations Development Programme (UNDP). (1994). *Human Security, Human Development Report*. New York: United Nations.

United Nations General Assembly (UNGA) (2009). "Global Health and Foreign Policy." A/ RES/63/33, 28 January. http://www.un.org/en/ga/search/view_doc.asp?symbol=A/RES/63/33.

United Nations General Assembly (UNGA) (2010). "Global Health and Foreign Policy." A/RES /64/108, 19 February. http://www.un.org/en/ga/search/view_doc.asp?symbol=A/RES/64/108.

United Nations General Assembly (UNGA) (2011). "Global Health and Foreign Policy." A/ RES/65/95, 10 February. http://www.un.org/en/ga/search/view_doc.asp?symbol=A/RES/65/95.

United Nations General Assembly (UNGA) (2012). "Global Health and Foreign Policy." A/RES /66/115, 24 February. http://www.un.org/en/ga/search/view_doc.asp?symbol=A/RES/66/115.

United Nations General Assembly (UNGA) (2013). "Global Health and Foreign Policy." A/RES /67/81, 14 March. http://www.un.org/en/ga/search/view_doc.asp?symbol=A/RES/67/81.

United Nations System Influenza Coordination (UNSIC) Asia-Pacific Regional Hub (2011). *Avian and Pandemic Influenza Related Programmes and Projects of the Inter-governmental Entities in Asia and the Pacific.* June. Bangkok: UNSIC.

Uppsala Conflict Data Program (UCPD) (2017). "UCDP Conflict Encyclopedia." Uppsala University. www.ucdp.uu.se.

Urdal, Henrik and Chi Primus Che (2013). "War and Gender Inequalities in Health: The Impact of Armed Conflict on Fertility and Maternal Mortality." *International Interactions* 39 (4): 489–510.

Vu, Tuong (2010). "Power, Politics and Accountability: Vietnam's Response to Avian Influenza." In Ian Scoones (ed.), *Avian Influenza: Science, Policy and Politics,* 93–130. London: Earthscan.

Weir, Lorna and Eric Mykhalovskiy (2010). *Global Public Health Vigilance: Creating a World on Alert.* New York: Routledge.

Wenham, Claire (2016). "Ebola Responsibility: Moving from Shared to Multiple Responsibilities." *Third World Quarterly* 37 (3): 436–451.

Whelan, Mary (2008). "Negotiating the International Health Regulations." Global Health Working Paper no. 1. Geneva: Graduate Institute.

WHO Western Pacific Regional Office (WPRO) (2005). "The Asia Pacific Strategy for Emerging Diseases." Manila: South-East Asia Regional Organization and Western Pacific Regional Organization for WHO.

WHO Western Pacific Regional Office (WPRO) (2006). *SARS: How a Global Epidemic Was Stopped.* Manila: World Health Organization for the Western Pacific Region.

WHO Western Pacific Regional Office (WPRO) (2010). *Asia Pacific Strategy for Emerging Diseases.* Manila: South-East Asia Regional Organization and Western Pacific Regional Organization for WHO.

WHO Western Pacific Regional Office (WPRO) (2012). *Securing Regional Health through APSED.* Progress Report. November. Manilla: WHO.

WHO Western Pacific Regional Office (WPRO) (2015). *Asia Pacific Strategy for Emerging Diseases Progress Report 2015.* Geneva: World Health Organization.

WHO Western Pacific Regional Office (WPRO) (2016). *Asia Pacific Strategy for Emerging Diseases and Public Health Emergencies.* WPR/RC67/9. Regional Committee Sixty-Seventh Session, 31 August. Manila: World Health Organization.

Wigley, Simon and Arzu Akkoyunlu-Wigley (2011). "The Impact of Regime Type on Health: Does Redistribution Explain Everything?" *World Politics* 63 (4): 647–677.

Wilsmore, Anthony, Anne Ancia, Elisabeth Dieleman, and Naushad Faiz (2010). "Outcome and Impact Assessment of the Global Response to the Avian Influenza Crisis 2005–2010." Luxembourg: Publications Office of the European Union.

Wipfli, Heather (2015). *The Global War on Tobacco: Mapping the World's First Public Health Treaty.* Baltimore: Johns Hopkins University Press.

World Bank (2016). "Heavily Indebted Poor Countries (HIPC) Initiative and Multilateral Debt Relief Initiative (MDRI)—Statistical Update." March. http://pubdocs.worldbank.org/en /1286146003908395/Statistical-Update-2015.pdf.

World Bank (2017). "World Bank Development Indicators." http://data.worldbank.org/indicator.

World Health Assembly (WHA) (1995). "Revision and Updating of the International Health Regulations." WHA48.7, 12 May. Geneva: World Health Organization.

World Health Assembly (WHA) (2001a). "Global Health Security: Epidemic Alert and Response." WHA54.14, 21 May. Geneva: World Health Organization.

World Health Assembly (WHA) (2001b). *Global Health Security—Epidemic Alert and Response*. Report by the Secretariat. A54/9, 2 April. Geneva: World Health Organization.

World Health Assembly (WHA) (2005). "Revision of the International Health Regulations." WHA58.3, 23 May. Geneva: World Health Organization.

World Health Assembly (WHA) (2006). "Application of the International Health Regulations (2005)." WHA59.2, 26 May 2006. Geneva: World Health Organization.

World Health Assembly (WHA) (2011). *Implementation of the International Health Regulations: Report of the Review Committee on the Functioning of the International Health Regulations (2005) in Relation to Pandemic (H1N1) 2009*. Report by the Director-General. A64/10, 5 May 2011. Geneva: World Health Organization.

World Health Assembly (WHA) (2016a). *Implementation of the International Health Regulations*. Report of the Review Committee on Second Extensions for Establishing National Public Health Capacities and on IHR Implementation. A68/22 Add.1, 27 March. Geneva: World Health Organization.

World Health Assembly (WHA) (2016b). *Implementation of the International Health Regulations (2005)*. Report of the Review Committee on the Role of the International Health Regulations (2005) in the Ebola Outbreak and Response. A69/21, 13 May. Geneva: World Health Organization.

World Health Organization (WHO) ([1948] 2009). *Constitution of the World Health Organization*. 47th ed. Geneva: World Health Organization.

World Health Organization (WHO) (2000). *A Framework for Global Outbreak Alert and Response*. WHO/CDS/CSR/2000.2. Geneva: World Health Organization.

World Health Organization (WHO) (2004). *World Health Organization Intergovernmental Working Group on Revision of the International Health Regulations: Summary Report of Regional Consultations*. A/IHR/IGWG/2, 14 September. Geneva: World Health Organization.

World Health Organization (WHO) (2005). *Revision of International Health Regulations, Report of the Third Regional Consultation, New Delhi, 27–29 January 2005*. New Delhi: Regional Office for South-East Asia.

World Health Organization (WHO) (2006). *The World Health Report 2006: Working Together for Health*. Geneva: World Health Organization.

World Health Organization (WHO) (2007a). "IHR: Areas of Work for Implementation." Geneva: World Health Organization.

World Health Organization (WHO) (2007b). *The World Health Report 2007: A Safer Future; Global Public Health Security in the 21st Century*. Geneva: World Health Organization.

World Health Organization (WHO) (2008). *International Health Regulations (2005)*. 2nd ed. Geneva: World Health Organization.

World Health Organization (WHO) (2010). "Guidance for the Use of Annex 2 of the International Health Regulations (2005)." WHO/HSE/IHR/2010.4. Geneva: World Health Organization.

World Health Organization (WHO) (2011). "H5N1 Avian Influenza: Timeline of Major Events." 7 November. http://www.who.int/influenza/human_animal_interface/avian_influenza/H5N1_avian_influenza_update.pdf.

World Health Organization (WHO) (2014). "Information to States Parties regarding Determination of Fulfilment of IHR National Core Capacity Requirements and Potential Extensions." Global Capacities Alert and Response. WHO/HSE/GCR/2014.9, January. Geneva: World Health Organization.

World Health Organization (WHO) (2015). "One Year into the Ebola Epidemic." January. http://www.who.int/csr/disease/ebola/one-year-report/introduction/en/.

World Health Organization (WHO) (2016a). "Progress Report on the Development of the WHO Health Emergencies Programme." 30 March. Geneva: World Health Organization.

World Health Organization (WHO) (2016b). *Joint External Evaluation Tool: International Health Regulations (2005)*. Geneva: World Health Organization.

World Health Organization (WHO) (2016c). "Global Strategy on Human Resources for Health: Workforce 2030." Geneva: World Health Organization.

World Health Organization (WHO) (2017a). "International Health Regulations (2005): Monitoring Framework, Global Health Observatory (GHO) Data Repository." Geneva: World Health Organization.

World Health Organization (WHO) (2017b). Table of Regional Averages for Key Indicators 2008, Global Health Expenditure Database. Geneva: World Health Organization.

World Health Organization (WHO) (2017c). "Life Expectancy by WHO Region, 2008: Global Health Observatory (GHO) Data Repository." Geneva: World Health Organization.

World Health Organization (WHO) (2017d). "Dengue and Severe Dengue." Factsheet. April. Geneva: World Health Organization. http://www.who.int/mediacentre/factsheets/fs117/en/.

World Health Organization (WHO) (2017e). "Nipah Virus Infection. Factsheet." Geneva: World Health Organization. http://www.who.int/csr/disease/nipah/en/.

World Health Organization (WHO) (2017f). "Dengue Control." http://www.who.int/denguecontrol/en/.

World Health Organization (WHO) (2017g). "WHO Guidelines on Ethical Issues in Public Health Surveillance." Geneva: World Health Organization.

Writing Committee of the Second World Health Organization Consultation on Clinical Aspects of Human Infection with Avian Influenza A (H5N1) Virus (2008). "Update on Avian Influenza A (H5N1) Virus Infection in Humans." *New England Journal of Medicine* 358: 261–273.

Writing Committee of the World Health Organization (WHO) Consultation on Human Influenza A/H5 (2005). "Avian Influenza A (H5N1) Infection in Humans." *New England Journal of Medicine* 353: 1374–1385.

Yoon, Sungwon (2010). "Ideas, Institutions, and Interests in the Global Governance of Epidemics in Asia." *Asia Pacific Journal of Public Health* 22 (3): 125–131.

Youde, Jeremy (2009). *Biopolitical Surveillance and Public Health in International Relations*. New York: Palgrave Macmillan.

Zacher, Mark W. and Tania J. Keefe (2008). *The Politics of Global Health Governance*. New York: Palgrave Macmillan.

Page numbers in *italics* indicate figures and tables.